D0502238

Seven Pillars of Health

Joseph
Christiano

SILOAM PRESS

Living in Health—Body, Mind and Spirit

SEVEN PILLARS OF HEALTH by Joseph Christiano
Published by Siloam Press
A part of Strang Communications Company
600 Rinehart Road
Lake Mary, Florida 32746
www.creationhouse.com

This book or parts thereof may not be reproduced in any form, stored in a
retrieval system or transmitted in any form by any means—electronic,
mechanical, photocopy, recording or otherwise—without prior written
permission of the publisher, except as provided by United States copyright
law.

Unless otherwise noted, all Scripture quotations are from the Holy Bible, New
International Version. Copyright © 1973, 1978, 1984, International Bible
Society. Used by permission.

Interior design by Karen Gonsalves

Incidents and persons portrayed in this volume are based on fact. Some names
and details have been changed and altered to protect the privacy of the
individuals to whom they refer. Any similarity between the names and stories
of individuals described in this book and individuals known to readers is
purely coincidental and not intentional.

Copyright © 2000 by Joseph Christiano
All rights reserved

Library of Congress Catalog Card Number: 00-104558
International Standard Book Number: 0-88419-693-3

This book is not intended to provide medical advice or to take the place of
medical advice and treatment from your personal physician. Readers are
advised to consult their own doctors or other qualified health professionals
regarding the treatment of their medical problems. Neither the publisher nor
the author takes any responsibility for any possible consequences from any
treatment, action or application of medicine, supplement, herb or preparation
to any person reading or following the information in this book. If readers are
taking prescription medications, they should consult with their physicians and
not take themselves off of medicines to start supplementation without the
proper supervision of a physician.

0 1 2 3 4 5 6 7 BVG 8 7 6 5 4 3 2 1
Printed in the United States of America

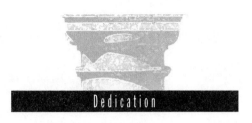

T his book is dedicated to Lori, my wife. She is the driving force behind me, the one who believes in me, the one who first suggested that I begin to write. She is my strength when I am weak, my joy when I am sad. She is my encourager, my best friend, my companion in and out of the business world, my soul mate. Thanks, babe. I love you!

Behind every successful man is a loving woman.

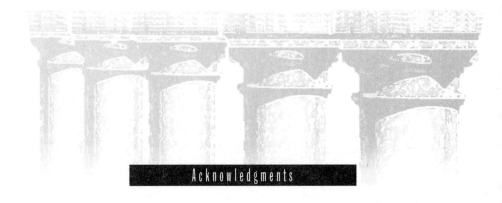

Acknowledgments

F or having a gift for detail, making sure every thought was clear and the directions exact, including countless late-night hours of e-mailing back and forth, compiling information, statistics and eventually finalizing the book content to meet our deadline, a task impossible alone—I give special thanks to Christina Williams, my blood type A ghostwriter.

A heartfelt "thank you" to all those at Siloam Press for seeing my vision and surrounding me with your expertise and encouragement. Special thanks go to Rick Nash and Gerry Bradley.

I cannot forget all the many people who played their role in my professional life, including clients, students and business associates who contributed to my expertise in health and fitness.

To fill these pages with encouragement and hope for people from all walks of life, I give an inexpressible "thank you" to God who allowed me all the years of experience and applied knowledge. Lending me the gifts and abilities to promote a balance in body, soul and spirit was in part His supernatural orchestration of my life's experiences that made it all possible. May all the praises be His.

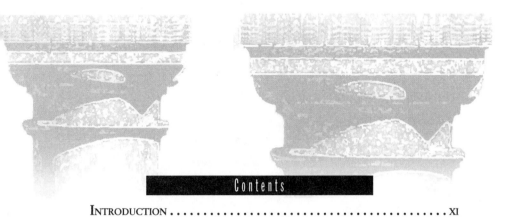

Contents

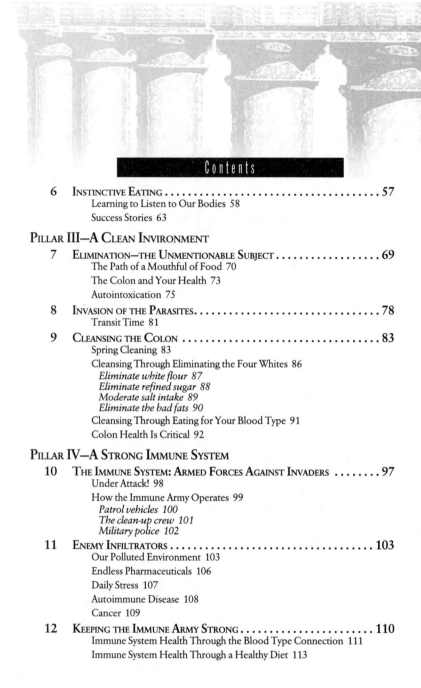

Contents

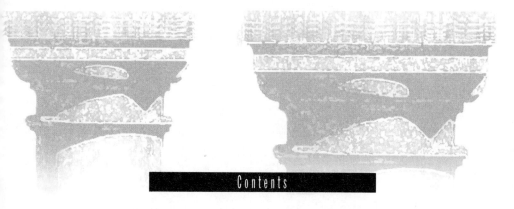

Contents

Contents

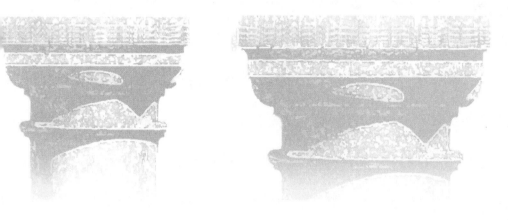

Do you not know that your body
is a temple of the Holy Spirit, who is in you,
whom you have received from God? You are not
your own; you were bought at a price.
Therefore honor God with your body.
—1 CORINTHIANS 6:19–20

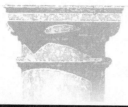

Superman, Mighty Mouse, Hercules—these were my childhood heroes. What kid didn't want to leap tall buildings in a single bound, run faster than a locomotive and bend steel with his bare hands? And who could surpass the likes of Mighty Mouse, with his bulging muscles and suave manner of rescuing damsels in distress? And what about Steve Reeves playing Hercules Unchained? Wow!

Looking back, I can see that I was destined to be a man of iron.

Maintaining a healthy body seemed to come naturally to me. Pumping iron, running, playing sports and staying physical—that just about sums up my life.

At the age of thirteen I learned how to lift weights in the spare bedroom of my parents' house. In high school I tried football, track and wrestling, but as I grew older my love for weight training won out. I could challenge myself to improve my physique without relying on others to make it happen.

Eventually I decided to turn my personal love into my profession, and I'm so glad I did! I started a gym in Orlando, Florida, and operated it in the late seventies and early eighties. Everyone was welcome, and I shared my expertise with all who asked. I enjoyed helping people who wanted to lose weight, put on some muscle or just to be fit.

As I continued in the health club business, I decided to switch my client focus from the competitive bodybuilder and powerlifter to the "deconditioned market." I guess that's a nice way to say "couch potatoes"—men and women who are not interested in becoming Mr. America or Miss America, but who have realized they need to do something about their overall condition or else be in serious trouble.

So after a couple of years privately training people and personally competing in national bodybuilding shows, I opened Body Redesigning, a private one-on-one fitness studio. It was the place to go to if you wanted to get in the best shape of your life. The concept was different from the typical health clubs where a person received nothing more than a lifetime membership card. At Body Redesigning, people enrolled in a ninety-day program, had the guidance of a personal trainer and access to a private training room.

As I continued building this new business of making fitness more personal, I ventured into training women for pageants. Several of the women I trained became swimsuit winners in the Miss USA, Miss America and Mrs. America pageants.

One day a phone call came with an offer I couldn't refuse—to be the corporate private trainer for Planet Hollywood. Needless to say, having a job in which I was flown in Lear jets, escorted to various destinations by limousine, accommodated in the most luxurious hotels in the world and fed in the fanciest restaurants was not hard to enjoy.

I trained the Planet Hollywood corporate executives as well as the celebrities. But among all the celebrities I worked with, Sylvester Stallone was my favorite. Maybe it was an Italian thing!

Though my position had wonderful perks and allowed me to see places like the French Riviera, Cancún and London, I felt drawn to help the Christian community learn about fitness. So I said good-bye to my Planet Hollywood days and started conducting Fitness

Introduction

and Fellowship classes with my wife, Lori, as well as writing material on exercise and nutrition.

Physical fitness has been my world for almost four decades. Over the years the Lord has allowed me the opportunity to learn about and experiment with diet and nutrition as well as exercise. I have seen it all and tried it all. And this book contains what I've learned through experience to be the best of the best.

It is my passion to serve as a conduit of information and services that help people become healthier and more energetic. I've always believed in maintaining and even improving health and fitness. And since I've passed the half-century mark, I've seen from a fresh perspective the need to keep our "temples" healthy so we can enjoy life as long as possible.

Our bodies are like temples with massive pillars holding up the superstructure. Our physical well-being is dependent upon the strength and condition of each pillar. If a pillar is cracked or crumbling, the temple is subject to collapse. But when well maintained, these pillars of health will defend us from sickness, disease and a breakdown in the quality of life.

Over the years I have discovered seven areas that need to be maintained in order to protect our health. These Seven Pillars of Health do not come with a lifetime guarantee. They must be continually kept up to assure their good condition. Plus, each Pillar is dependent upon the strength and condition of the others. When one cracks or crumbles, the others are weakened.

Let's take a look at these Seven Pillars of Health in order to understand the important role they play in protecting our health.

- *Weight management*—We have all struggled with that one, haven't we? But did you know that weight is not just an appearance issue, but also a health issue? And weight is more than a number on a scale—it has to do with body composition, too.

Seven Pillars of Health

- *Diet*—Don't we hate that word! That's because we associate it with punishing and depriving ourselves. But diet also refers to the type of foods we choose to eat. If we eat correctly for our biochemistry, we never have to diet!

- *A clean invironment*—The word *invironment* was coined by Dr. Albert Zake: "While the environment is the atmosphere and surroundings in which we live, the 'invironment' is the atmosphere and surroundings inside us."[1] We may not realize it, but our diet of processed and fast foods has been devastating to our colons. I know, the condition of our colons is not a subject we talk much about, but it's time to start! We need to cleanse our invironments of the toxins that are undermining our health.

- *A strong immune system*—The best defense against sickness and disease is a strong immune system. Perhaps you didn't realize that we can do many things to actually strengthen our defenses so they can successfully fight viruses and bacteria. The best way to get well is never to get sick!

- *Exercise*—Uh-oh, you knew this was coming. Yes, exercise has now been tied directly to the state of our health. Exercise is not just toning up and strengthening anymore. It's a tonic for joint health, heart health and just about every other kind of health.

- *Rest and relaxation*—This is the fun pillar. We all need to discover simple ways to de-stress and relax. Rest is essential for our health. Did you know that our bodies actively work to restore our health while we sleep? Missing sleep can weaken our overall condition.

- *Anti-aging strategies*—Perhaps you went to sleep and awakened middle-aged! Then you will want to pay attention

Introduction

to these anti-aging strategies. We no longer have to "look forward" to a season of debilitation and pain in our later years. There are steps we can take now to bring vigor and health to our senior years.

Are you ready to journey forward to improve your health, strengthen and tone your muscles and enjoy life to its fullest? I'll try to make the journey as simple as possible. I love to dispel the mystery and confusion that obscures the road to fitness, so your chances of being successful will be as great as possible.

One more thing—I have spent many years pursuing physical fitness. All my efforts have been directed toward being healthier, stronger and in the best form possible. But a day came when something inside me cried out, "What's it all for?"

As you pursue a greater quality of life physically, remember that God is the giver of life, both physical and spiritual. We cannot be complete without being healthy in body, soul and spirit. Give God a place in your life. In fact, give Him your life itself. I came to understand that's the only way to find out what it's all for.

Then you will have a surpassing reason to be a faithful caretaker of your body, which He has so graciously given you.

Now, let's find out how to strengthen our Seven Pillars of Health.

Weight Management

*Like a city whose walls are
broken down is a man who
lacks self-control.*
—Proverbs 25:28

PILLAR ONE

1

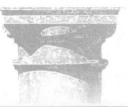

EATING, EMOTIONS AND ITALIANS

In April 1981 I had my "Kodak moment." I had just picked up a packet of photos I had developed, and I was eagerly looking through them. I stopped instantly when I came upon a picture of myself. There I was—all 305 pounds of me. Did I really look like that? I just couldn't believe it.

First I went into shock. Then I was overcome with embarrassment.

Two questions whirled through my mind: *How in the world did I get into this condition? And how in the world was I going to get out of it?*

The first question was easy to answer. It wasn't as though I had gone to sleep weighing 220 and awakened the next morning weighing 305. Somehow, little by little, day by day, I had eaten my way to 305.

The irony of the whole thing was that I was in the fitness business! But something had gone haywire.

The second question haunted me. What in the world could I do? One option was to panic, latch onto the latest fad diet and go for the quick fix. But the results would be temporary at best, and I knew it. I would end right back at 305—or higher.

Seven Pillars of Health

In order to truly and permanently get out of my heavy condition, I had to take a serious look inside. I knew enough to realize that the weight was just a symptom. So what was the real problem? I decided to go back to my childhood to see if I could discover something in my upbringing that could be linked to my dilemma.

Food and Family—the Italian Way

My Italian mother just loved to feed her family—doing that was her pride and joy. I was raised on homemade Italian food, and all our meals were made from scratch. So it's hard to think of anything any better than that!

I remember coming home from school in the middle of the winter, and even a block away from the house I could smell an aroma so overwhelming that I would almost float to the kitchen door. As I went in, there before me on the kitchen table were twelve pans of the most fabulous, scrumptious and delicious homemade bread on the face of the earth. Down the sides of each loaf streamed rivulets of melting butter. The loaves just screamed for me to dig in.

As I stood there with my tongue hanging out, my mother would ask proudly, "Joey, would you like a piece of bread?" Before I could answer, she would hack off a wedge about three inches thick, slather it with butter and thrust it into my hands. Every day we ate her homemade dishes—pasta, ravioli, gnocchi, chicken cacciatore, pigs in the blanket (cabbage rolls)—plus that homemade bread.

As I thought about this, I got a better picture of how large a role food played in my younger years. I also recalled our eating behavior, which was determined by my father. He was a man of few words, but when he spoke, we listened—or else! At the supper table he had only one rule: "Take all you want, but eat all you take." Did I grow up in a great world, or what? It didn't take long for us four kids to learn how to pack it away.

Even my only sister, Judy, abided by the rule. At age sixteen she

Eating, Emotions and Italians

was able to eat sixteen pigs in the blanket at one sitting—yet she was the size of Olive Oyl. My brothers, Ronny and Bob, would never take second place to their sister—and were known to consume thirty ravioli each at one sitting. So they too learned how to abide by the infamous rule.

I think my very best performance at the supper table occurred one Thanksgiving when I devoured the complete traditional dinner with every side dish you can imagine— plus two pounds of Ma's home-made pasta. Then I ate desserts—a couple of pieces of pumpkin pie and pecan pie—and chased it all down with a quart of eggnog.

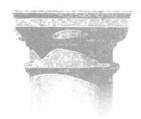

My folks would say proudly to my aunt and uncle, "You should have seen how much Joey ate yesterday! You would never believe it." And my aunt and uncle would always respond, "God bless Joey. He's a good boy!"

So, do you think I may have found the answer to my first question? Yes, I realized how I got this way. Knowing that was the beginning, but there was more than one piece to the puzzle.

EMOTIONAL EATING

IT IS COMMON in many Italian families (and I'm sure other families as well) for everyone to talk gaily about those who eat big. The topic of conversation was always food at my aunt and uncle's house. All my relatives heard about how much I could eat. Why, a big eater like me made the front page in the *Italian Gazette!* My folks would say proudly to my aunt and uncle, "You should have seen how much Joey ate yesterday! You would never believe it." And my aunt and uncle would always respond, "God bless Joey. He's a good boy!"

So, I would get a pat on the back for eating like a pig.

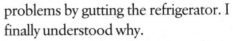

Seven Pillars of Health

When I was a kid I burned up all those calories playing. But at the age of thirty-one I weighed 305 pounds. At that time I was also struggling with some personal problems that brought on a lot of emotional stress. My self-esteem dove to an all-time low, and I began not liking myself. So I had unconsciously coped with my emotional problems by gutting the refrigerator. I finally understood why.

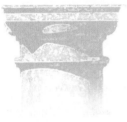

Once I realized there was a connection between eating and feeling worthwhile, I could better understand how to fix my problem.

Isn't the connection between body and soul fascinating? Stored in my mental memory bank was a feeling of praise, a good stroke, a pat on the back: "Joey's a good boy. God bless him." And all I had to do to get that stroke at my lowest time was to eat. Subconsciously, eating soothed me and eased my emotional pain. I ate a large volume of food because the more I ate, the better I felt about myself, about others—and about life itself!

Once I realized there was a connection between eating and feeling worthwhile, I could better understand how to fix my problem. Then I could look at that photograph and see my overweight condition as a symptom of emotional and psychological trouble. Had I continued to deal with it by eating, it would likely have led to health problems.

After analyzing the eating behaviors to which I was accustomed, I realized that over the years I had lost focus of the purpose of food—to nourish the body. Instead, food had become a method of coping with my personal life issues. I was used to seeing food as a friend who met my emotional needs. Instead, food should have been my servant—providing the nutrition I needed for the demands placed on my physical body by everything I was going through. But because I

Eating, Emotions and Italians

was an emotional eater, the value of food as a means of nourishing my body became blurred. Just like the subtle loss of eyesight over one's lifetime, my relationship with food had become out of focus—and I finally realized I needed glasses.

It was clear that I needed to turn the unhealthy way I was living into a healthy, well-balanced and fit life. In order for me to be set free from this emotional stronghold, I had to make some changes and establish some boundaries.

Boundaries and Eating Disorders

Boundaries are necessary in every area of our lives. For instance, marriages need boundaries that allow us time with our spouses as well as time alone. If we disagree with our spouse, boundaries keep us from injuring the other person with angry words. Boundaries are vitally important for our children, too. Our kids need freedom to grow through experience, but that freedom must be accompanied by structure for guidance and for proper emotional, spiritual and physical development.

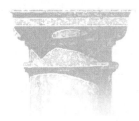

Eating disorders are often connected back to these invasions of boundaries.

Boundaries help us develop better control over our lives, whether in marriage, family, business, our relationship with God, exercise or eating.

The whole focus is to develop a more balanced lifestyle. But when emotional, physical, psychological, sexual and even intellectual boundaries have been consistently ignored or invaded, for instance as in a childhood experience of abuse, then our experience is one of invasion of boundaries, not respect for them. A person with such a background hasn't had the experience of setting boundaries that others won't cross.

Eating disorders are often connected back to these invasions of boundaries. If a person has no way to stop the invasions, then he or she experiences helplessness, despair and a sense of worthlessness. Sometimes people didn't know how to set boundaries when they were young. Perhaps a young girl was humiliated by her brother's reading her diary to his friends, but she never told him the consequences of his doing something like that again. She was wounded, but she never dealt with the wound. Emotional issues can turn into health issues. One result of not setting boundaries is an eating disorder.

Without boundaries, one can eat for emotional relief, as I did. I ate vast amounts of food to feel value, comfort and worth. This kind of compulsive eating stems from a lack of control, a negligence in setting boundaries. The choice to eat, in my case, was based on self-medication rather than physical hunger. Consequently, compulsive overeaters will eat whenever and whatever they please. Since they never establish boundaries, they don't know how to stop eating when they're full.

Enough has no meaning to the bulimic either. The compulsive overeater will stop when the stomach is so full that it is distended. But the bulimic will eat, then vomit and perhaps eat some more. Again, there are no limits.

Anorexics behave in an opposite matter. They will virtually starve themselves to death in search of relief from emotional pain. They have not set boundaries—in this case, ones that say they must eat for nourishment. They have no boundaries that declare they are not allowed to neglect eating or to eat too little. Their situation can get so serious that death seems to be spiritual bliss and the final act of protecting themselves from their emotional pain.

Many of us have areas in our eating behaviors in which we have set no boundaries for ourselves. Some people are sugarholics and will sacrifice their health to satisfy their sweet tooth. Others eat too much salt; they will overeat salty foods such as potato chips. I know soda drinkers who drink way too much soda because they like the feel of the fizz in their throats. All these excesses are the result of not setting boundaries.

Certainly the reasons people have these disorders are vast and complex, stemming from sexual abuse to invasion of privacy to a lack of power over their lives. I am neither a psychologist nor an expert in this area, but for decades I have observed people working on weight management. They try the widely available self-help programs, such as support groups and dieting organizations. These resources are good. But if people become dependent on the *system* and still have not dealt with the *issue behind the lack of boundaries,* then they become vulnerable when they leave that support organization. Often they go back to their old ways because they were operating on external rules rather than internal boundaries.

Emotional disorders can be manifested through bad eating habits. People who have been violated feel unworthy, of no value. Coming to grips with who they really are will make a difference. I have come to believe that the perfect relief from pain and inappropriate invasions of boundaries—whether by caretakers, parents, siblings or strangers—is an acceptance of God's love for us.

God gives us freedom, but we don't experience that freedom because we live out of our past, out of our unresolved issues. So we don't feel worthy of God's love or the love of others. But God accepts us as we are. He forgives us when we ask Him. He restores us emotionally. That's who He is. Really connecting with the truth that God loves us can free us. If we can understand how God accepts us as we are, then we can feel accepted and of value. And that releases a lot of baggage.

Once we have this new view of ourselves, our eyes are opened to see the abuse we were causing ourselves by our bad eating habits.

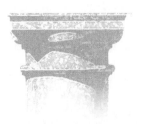

When we exert self-control by setting boundaries, we are released from the cycle of feeling like a bad person when we gain a few pounds.

That sets in motion the desire for boundaries. Then, with God's help, we can successfully exert self-control and set boundaries. And self-control is necessary for victory over emotional eating problems.

Remember, boundaries are not rules. Rules tell you exactly what you can eat and when. Once you have set up boundaries in your eating, you can choose to have something special at certain times without that urge taking over and becoming an everyday habit. Boundaries set us free.

Self-Control Is Freedom

Self-control is the healthful regulation of our desires and appetites. Self-control prevents excess. When we exert self-control by setting boundaries, we are released from the cycle of feeling like a bad person when we gain a few pounds. We won't have the false guilt that comes with always going on and off diets. We won't feel like a failure.

As human beings, we have a nature that leans toward wrong-doing. Think of what people would be like without self-control! Though we don't like to admit it, dangerous desires dwell within our hearts. When self-control is strong, we are safe. But when it is weak, we are weak as well—and vulnerable to self-destructive behavior.

God's creation is to be enjoyed. We should enjoy eating—the tastes, the textures, the fun of creating exciting dishes, the socializing around a meal. But because our desires have been corrupted, God's intended enjoyments of eating can become our master instead of our servant.

Eating, Emotions and Italians

Self-control holds us in bounds, not in bondage. Self-control gives us power over our lives. It allows us to put boundaries in place, boundaries that help us achieve our desires and dreams.

A Personal Decision
to Set Up Boundaries

REVIEWING MY UPBRINGING helped me come to grips with the reality that food could not solve any of my emotional problems, regardless of what emotion I might be facing at the time. I also realized that when I got emotionally excited or stimulated, I would immediately turn to food.

For me, not having boundaries allowed food to become my enemy. I needed to put in place some boundaries that would prevent my emotions from becoming my reason for eating food. I also recognized that I needed to regain a connection with the human race and reestablish a balance of sound mind and emotion. I felt like a second-rate citizen. Weighing 305, I felt like a pig, I dressed like a pig and I certainly ate like a pig. So, in my own mind, I somehow had to feel human again.

What did I do? First, I changed my food selections. Believe me, my Kodak moment gave me all the motivation I needed to do that. Soon I started noticing changes in my appearance just from eating different foods. The more I experimented with making proper food selections, the better the physical results were.

Next, I changed my training program by adding aerobic training to my progressive strength training. I was eating for only one purpose—to meet the demands made on my physical body and to reach my goals.

Then, I dealt with my emotional attachment to eating by making the choice to deal with each emotion as it came along. Instead of eating to medicate my feelings, I listened to music, exercised, prayed or got together with people who would make me laugh.

Along the way I discovered more about myself and what I enjoyed. I did whatever it took to no longer eat my way through my emotions. Eating lost its role as a means of coping with my emotional and psychological battles.

Finally, I was putting everything in perspective. I had a grip on my emotions about eating, and I felt an overwhelming sense of freedom. Eventually, I began liking myself again.

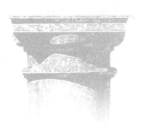

I define victory as having my boundaries in place and honoring them with self-control.

Developing a balanced mind, having self-control and staying focused is the baseline. It would be nice to have someone come along and pick up all the broken pieces of our lives, but that won't happen. We have to do it ourselves, and it all starts within.

In that April of 1981, I promised myself that I was never going to get out of control like that again. I owed myself a better quality of life, and I was bound and determined to get it.

As I followed my boundaries, I started losing body fat and gaining muscularity. Soon I looked completely different. My friends saw my progress and encouraged me to compete in bodybuilding. In December 1981, at 220 pounds, I won the Mr. Florida title. In 1982 I took first runner-up in the Mr. USA contest and fourth runner-up in Mr. America.

I had dropped 85 pounds in just eight months.

Amazingly, my goal had not been one of those titles or even bodybuilding itself. My primary goal was never again to be in the condition in which I found myself that day in April. And ever since, I have had absolutely no problem maintaining my weight. As a matter of fact, that has been the easiest part of the journey.

Eating, Emotions and Italians

Applying Personal Boundaries

Dɪᴅ I ǫᴜɪᴛ being an emotional eater? No. That's deeply ingrained in me. The difference is that now I am aware of it, and I know how to address it. I still have to remind myself to put up boundaries. I don't know if I will ever gain complete victory over this problem—that is, if victory is defined as never desiring to eat for emotional reasons. I define victory as having my boundaries in place and honoring them with self-control.

HEALTH FACT BOX

If I find myself reaching for food as a way to deal with emotions, I now make these adjustments:
1. I stop eating (sometimes before I start). Drinking water (especially sparkling water) instead of eating helps me.
2. I remind myself that I'm not hungry.
3. I get physical as soon as possible by taking a walk, training or doing some kind of exercise or exertion.

Knowledge and how we apply it make all the difference between success and failure. I came to see emotional eating as an enemy to my physical and mental health. I found that staying focused on the type of lifestyle I preferred to maintain was a key for helping me overcome the out-of-control urges to eat, which were caused by emotions. I have determined to turn this problem into the fuel necessary for me to work harder at being in balance.

Seven Pillars of Health

If you struggle with emotional eating as I do, then I wholly encourage you to do likewise. Instead of using it as an excuse to stay as you are, turn it into the motivation to be an overcomer. Your worst enemy can become your greatest strength if you just decide to take that first step toward change.

2

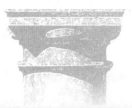

Weight Management

WEIGHT AND
THE PERFECT BODY

W hat constitutes the perfect female body?"

That was the question I asked 250 women at a recent Wellness Conference for Women in Orlando, Florida.

The perfect female would be five feet, eight inches tall, have long, slender legs and a flat tummy. At least, that's what some women said. Others claimed she would be taller, yet with a full figure. Still others felt that the petite figure was the perfect one.

After I heard the opinions of the women in the audience, I described the perfect female: "She's a woman five feet, two inches tall, weighing 185 pounds and with 36 percent body fat."

I think the people in the next room probably heard the collective gasp.

Without an explanation, I pressed on to what constituted a perfect male body. Responses were rapidly shouted out.

"Six feet tall with wide shoulders and a firm lower body," came one. "A muscular chest and arms," another yelled out.

"Hmmm," I responded. "Actually, the perfect man is four feet, eleven inches tall and weighs 95 pounds."

Of course, everyone thought I was nuts. My descriptions were nowhere near theirs.

Finally, I had mercy on my audience. "The perfect female body is actually a real woman. She happens to be a world champion cold-water swimmer who swam the frigid waters of the English Channel..."

I heard a collective sigh of relief.

"...and she has the perfect body for her sport. Her high percentage of body fat serves as the ideal insulation for protecting her from the cold waters and makes her more buoyant and able to stay afloat in the water.

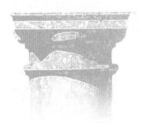

So, if this obsession to lose weight has been around for decades, why are people still struggling with taking it off and keeping it off?

"My description of the man under five feet tall and weighing less than 100 pounds is also a real person," I continued. "He was a world champion horse jockey with a body perfect for his sport. Having a body short in stature and light in weight made for the perfect horse rider."

Perhaps the man and woman I described don't represent the perfect male and female bodies to you. They certainly didn't to my audience that day. But I bet that if I asked you about the perfect male and female bodies, you would have images in mind. Where do those images come from?

THE IMAGE OF PERFECTION

WE'VE ALL BEEN affected by advertisements, movies and television. Our images of perfection usually match the bodies of the stars we see on TV and magazine covers. Both the high-fashion modeling industry and Hollywood hold first place in the influence department because of the tremendous presence they maintain.

Many females—adults, teenagers and even preteens—have low self-esteem and don't like themselves just because they believe their bodies do not match up with those being displayed in the fashion magazines or on TV. The media's message is so strong that if we are not grounded with good information, we can be psychologically disabled—particularly if we cannot get control of our weight.

Ever since the diet craze of the eighties, people have been trying to attain a perfect body by losing weight. A multibillion dollar industry has been created around this national obsession. Thousands of lotions, potions and pills call out to the frustrated dieter, promising a perfect body. Just look at the magazines in your supermarket checkout lane. You can read about several new diet plans in the few minutes while you're in line. It's total insanity.

Women secretly wrap themselves in plastic to sweat away inches. Pageant contestants spend money on body wrap sessions—all to lose weight. I know a bit about the gimmicks because I have helped women who compete in pageants go from a size twelve down to a size eight in ninety days. I have trained swimsuit winners in the Miss USA, Miss America and Mrs. America Pageants.

So, if this obsession to lose weight has been around for decades, why are people still struggling with taking it off and keeping it off?

LACKING THE RIGHT INFORMATION

I BELIEVE PEOPLE struggle with dieting and weight because of a lack of knowledge. There is a difference between losing weight and losing fat. Once we understand that, we will understand the statistics that show as many as 95 percent of people who diet gain it all back within three years.[1] With all the diet plans that have come and gone throughout the years, isn't it amazing that there is only a 20 percent success rate? Maybe diets are not the answer.

Seven Pillars of Health

The outward appearance is what drives most people to lose weight. That's what drove the pageant contestants. If people will follow healthy guidelines for weight management and the other Pillars of Health, a pleasing cosmetic result will be the by-product.

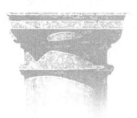

This yo-yo system of weight management is not only unhealthy, but it also brings with it feelings of guilt and failure that contribute to giving up.

For the longest time people have lost their battle with the bulge. Many people lose weight, then gain it right back. Did you know that this yo-yo syndrome can cause cracks in the Pillar of Weight Management because it interferes with the normal metabolic process? Zipping up and down on the scale can cause a person's ideal set point, or the balance between calorie consumption and calorie expenditure, to become out of kilter. When there is a constant fluctuation of weight gain and then weight loss, the body returns to a low set point where it will burn less calories. It feels as if it's going into a starvation mode, so as a survival mechanism, it conserves calories. That causes weight gain.

My clients who have lost weight and then gained it back again testify to the frustration and discouragement this brings. This yo-yo system of weight management is not only unhealthy, but it also brings with it feelings of guilt and failure that contribute to giving up. This emotional and mental strain eventually creates low-self esteem and unnecessary stress.

Yet most bulge fighters will grab at anything that comes along. But "anything that comes along" may be the newest star's diet excitingly attested to in the supermarket tabloid. People often take unhealthy approaches to managing their weight because they haven't identified the sources that influence their decisions.

Weight and the Perfect Body

For some, the source is childhood habits, such as I've described from my own life. Others make decisions influenced by social trends and the quick-fix mind-set. Still others haphazardly grab at straws—or whatever diet is in vogue at the moment.

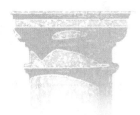

Even though we are bombarded with a tremendous emphasis on looks, weight and style, the answer isn't just winning the fight against the social trends or fashions, for they will always influence us. The answer is getting a better understanding of our own situation, then doing something about it.

I believe how much you weigh is not as important as the quality of your weight.

My main concern is that people have healthier and more energetic lives. Shaking off the "body beautiful" mind-set and taking on a more serious attitude toward weight management can lead not only to good health, but also to vitality and a new zest for life.

WEIGHT—FRIEND OR FOE?

AM I SAYING that weight management is not important? No, I believe it is important. But there's more to weight management than that number on the scale you dread waking up to every morning.

Why is the amount you weigh important? Unless you have to weigh in every day to keep your job, why stress yourself over it? We may not have to, but we do, don't we? And if you are conscious of your weight at all times, then you probably looked better at a lower weight once—and you're trying to get back there.

I believe how much you weigh is not as important as the *quality* of your weight. The real question is, What is your weight revealing about you? Are you in shape or not? What is your body composition, and how do you feel?

Seven Pillars of Health

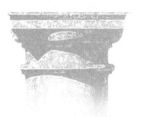

If you think you just have to lose a few pounds to look the way you want, then I want to issue you a challenge: Focus on the condition of your weight instead of the number on the scale.

Maintaining a lower percentage of body fat is more critical to your health than the number on the scale. When you lose body fat, you lose weight. But if you're only looking at weight, you can lose water weight and muscle and show weight loss, but that's not healthy.

Over the years, not only have I pursued a healthier standard of weight management in my own life, but I have also assisted hundreds of other people along this bumpy journey. In over three decades of work in health and fitness, I have discovered two very revealing realities regarding weight management: First, the measuring tape tells all; and second, the mirror never lies.

Let me ask you something scary: Have you taken a good look at yourself in the mirror lately? If you are like most people, looking into the mirror can be a traumatic experience, particularly if you have struggled to get your weight under control. But if you have the courage to look into the mirror, then you are ready for the first step toward making the necessary changes in your body.

When you look in the mirror, notice the condition of your body, not the weight. Take your measurements and see how your clothes fit. These are better standards to use than weight.

Most of us can be far too critical of our looks, and ultimately we become our own worse judge. Remember, the mirror is your best friend—one you can trust because it will never lie to you. If you can deal with its truthfulness, you have hope.

In our quest to maintain a healthy body weight, we will discover there is much more to it than meets the eye (when looking in the

Weight and the Perfect Body

mirror!). We will explore a broader view that will help you to gain control of your weight forever. By maintaining the correct preventative measures, the Pillar of Weight Management can remain a support column for the rest of your life.

Weight, Genetics and Body Composition

THE "PERFECT" MAN and woman I described to my conference audience had the best shape and composition for their sports. Yet, they weren't the shapes and sizes most people want. So the question is, Can we always have what we want? If that jockey had wanted to be a basketball player, he may have been out of luck. We have to work with what we have, don't we?

If you want to look like the model on the cover of *Cosmopolitan*, but you're five feet, two inches tall and weigh 160 pounds, and the model is five feet, eleven inches tall and weighs 130 pounds, good luck! You'll live in constant frustration, and a sense of failure will be your constant companion. We have to keep our desires within the parameters of our genetics.

My wife, Lori, did some modeling for a while. But she discovered that at five foot, seven inches tall, she was too short for runway modeling and too tall to model as a shorter person. Since she couldn't add or subtract inches to her genetically prescribed height, she had to settle for being a perfume model—but a beautiful one at that!

All of us have a potential we can reach based on our genetics, based on what we have been given. But it won't be somebody else's potential. Weight is part of genetics; sometimes we can't do anything about being too heavy or too thin. A large-framed person will never be petite.

Each of us has been given so much clay to work with. What we do with that clay is our responsibility. We do have control over body composition—whether we're fit or not. And that requires lifestyle and behavior changes.

If you think you just have to lose a few pounds to look the way you want, then I want to issue you a challenge: Focus on the condition of your weight instead of the number on the scale. Body weight is not important. What is important is the lean weight vs. the fat weight.

I have had many clients tell me the particular weight they were trying to reach. I would then ask, "Would you feel all right if you looked as though you weighed that particular number, but actually weighed more?" Their expressions usually went blank at that point because they had never thought it was possible to look lighter than they weighed.

You see, when we are fit, we may weigh more but look much better. So the number on the scale is less important than the fitness of the body standing on the scale.

Becoming fit is a smarter way to manage weight. Giving regular attention to the body's health and condition throughout the years will prevent a serious health condition called obesity. Understanding the health issues related to weight management will give us a better chance to win the fight against this enemy of our health.

3

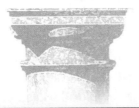

Weight Management

WEIGHT AND
YOUR HEALTH

One in three, or 58 million, American adults aged twenty through seventy-four are overweight.[1] Obesity is associated with nearly 822 deaths per day in America and costs the country more than $240 billion in obesity-related illnesses.[2] "Only smoking exceeds obesity in its contribution to total mortality rates in the United States. The nation can no longer afford to ignore obesity as a major medical problem," says Dr. William Dietz, director of Nutrition and Physical Activity for Disease Control and Prevention.[3]

Being overweight and physically inactive account for more than 300,000 premature deaths each year in the United States, second only to tobacco-related deaths. "Obesity and overweight are linked to the nation's number one killer—heart disease—as well as diabetes and other chronic conditions," says Jeffrey P. Koplan, director of the Centers for Disease Control (CDC).[4] Besides increasing the risks for heart disease and diabetes, obesity increases the risk of developing high blood pressure, stroke, gallbladder disease and cancer of the colon, prostate and breast.[5]

Sadly, since this condition exists among the adults in America, our children have become victims of it as well. The American lifestyle of inactivity has played a devastating role on the children of our country. Now, 11 percent of our children are overweight or obese.[6] Research has shown that 60 percent of overweight five- to ten-year-old children have at least one risk factor for heart disease, hyperlipidemia and elevated blood pressure or insulin levels.[7]

I can't tell you how many times I have counseled men in their late thirties and mid-forties who are recovering from recent heart attacks who have told me they wished they would have listened to all the advice they received—including losing excess weight—prior to their heart attack.

Yet the October 13, 1999, issue of *JAMA* showed that two-thirds of adults attempting to lose weight or keep from gaining it would rather take the weight-loss lotions, potions and pills than to follow sound, sensible guidelines that have the best chance of producing long-lasting results.[8] Without definite lifestyle changes, all the fad diets will only provide temporary results at best. The weight will keep coming back.

Studies show that an obese person generally dies prematurely, deals with heart disease for upwards of twelve to fifteen years and has more trips to the hospital—and therefore more medical bills.[9] Statistics indicate that an obese person can actually expect to add twenty quality years to his or her life simply by losing the excess weight.[10]

WHO IS AT RISK?

PERHAPS YOU WONDER if the extra fat you may be carrying is affecting you. Let's look at some ways to determine that.

The standards for measuring obesity or being overweight have changed in the last years. One way to determine obesity today is to use the body-mass index (BMI), which is a method of comparing height to weight.

Body Mass Index Chart

Weight (lbs.)	4'10"	4'11"	5'0"	5'1"	5'2"	5'3"	5'4"	5'5"	5'6"	5'7"	5'8"	5'9"	5'10"	5'11"	6'0"	6'1"	6'2"	6'3"	6'4"
100	21	20	20	19	18	18	17	17	16	16	15	15	14	14	14	13	13	13	12
105	22	21	21	20	19	19	18	17	17	16	16	16	15	15	14	14	13	13	13
110	23	22	21	21	20	19	19	18	18	17	17	16	16	15	15	15	14	14	13
115	24	23	22	22	21	20	20	19	19	18	17	17	17	16	16	15	15	14	14
120	25	24	23	23	22	21	21	20	19	19	18	18	17	17	16	16	15	15	15
125	26	25	24	24	23	22	21	21	20	20	19	18	18	17	17	16	16	16	15
130	27	26	25	25	24	23	22	22	21	20	20	19	19	18	18	17	17	16	16
135	28	27	26	26	25	24	23	22	22	21	21	20	19	19	18	18	17	17	16
140	29	28	27	26	26	25	24	23	23	22	21	21	20	20	19	18	18	17	17
145	30	29	28	27	27	26	25	24	23	23	22	21	21	20	20	19	19	18	18
150	31	30	29	28	27	27	26	25	24	23	23	22	22	21	20	20	19	19	18
155	32	31	30	29	28	27	27	26	25	24	24	23	22	22	21	20	20	19	19
160	33	32	31	30	29	28	27	27	26	25	24	24	23	22	22	21	21	20	19
165	34	33	32	31	30	29	28	27	27	26	25	24	24	23	22	22	21	21	20
170	36	34	33	32	31	30	29	28	27	27	26	25	24	24	23	22	22	21	21
175	37	35	34	33	32	31	30	29	28	27	27	26	25	24	24	23	22	22	21
180	38	36	35	34	33	32	31	30	29	28	27	27	26	25	24	24	23	23	22
185	39	37	36	35	34	33	32	31	30	29	28	27	27	26	25	24	24	23	23
190	40	38	37	36	35	34	33	32	31	30	29	28	27	27	26	25	24	24	23
195	41	39	38	37	36	35	33	32	31	31	30	29	28	27	27	26	25	24	24

Body Mass Index Chart

Weight (lbs.)	4'10"	4'11"	5'0"	5'1"	5'2"	5'3"	5'4"	5'5"	5'6"	5'7"	5'8"	5'9"	5'10"	5'11"	6'0"	6'1"	6'2"	6'3"	6'4"
200	42	40	39	38	37	36	34	33	32	31	30	30	29	28	27	26	26	25	24
205	43	41	40	39	38	36	35	34	33	32	31	30	29	29	28	27	26	26	25
210	44	43	41	40	39	37	36	35	34	33	32	31	30	29	28	27	27	26	26
215	45	44	42	41	39	38	37	36	35	34	33	32	31	30	29	28	28	27	26
220	46	45	43	42	40	39	38	37	36	34	33	32	32	31	30	29	28	27	27
225	47	46	44	43	41	40	39	38	36	35	34	33	32	31	31	30	29	28	27
230	48	47	45	44	42	41	40	38	37	36	35	34	33	32	31	30	30	29	28
235	49	48	46	45	43	42	40	39	38	37	36	35	34	33	32	31	30	29	29
240	50	49	47	46	44	43	41	40	39	38	37	35	34	33	33	32	31	30	29
245	51	50	48	47	45	43	42	41	40	38	37	36	35	34	33	32	32	31	30
250	52	51	49	48	46	44	43	42	40	39	38	37	36	35	34	33	32	31	30
255	53	52	50	49	47	45	44	43	41	40	39	37	36	35	34	33	32	32	31
260	54	53	51	50	48	46	45	44	42	41	40	38	37	36	35	34	33	32	32
265	56	54	52	51	49	47	46	44	43	42	41	39	38	37	36	35	34	33	32
270	57	55	53	51	50	48	46	45	44	42	41	40	39	38	37	36	35	34	33
275	58	56	54	52	50	49	47	46	44	43	42	41	39	38	37	36	35	34	34
280	59	57	55	53	51	50	48	47	45	44	43	41	40	39	38	37	36	35	34
285	60	58	56	54	52	51	49	48	46	45	43	42	41	40	39	38	37	36	35
290	61	59	57	55	53	51	50	48	47	45	44	43	42	41	39	38	37	36	35
300	63	61	59	57	55	53	52	50	49	47	46	44	43	42	41	40	39	38	37

Weight and Your Health

According to this chart, a person who is five feet, eight inches tall and weighs 140 pounds would have a BMI of 21. A BMI of 19 to 24.9 is considered to be within the normal range, while a BMI reading of 25 to 29.9 is considered to be overweight. Any reading over 30 is considered obese. Researchers who use this standard estimate that more than one-half of the adult America population is either obese or overweight![11] This approach does not factor in the individual's muscle development or lean muscle mass.

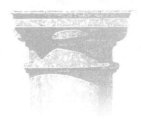

However, in my opinion, using just height and weight is simplifying it too much. Too many times I have seen men or women virtually panic over what the scale reads when, in fact, the scale is the worst and most inaccurate method of monitoring weight.

The scale tells us nothing about the quality or condition of weight. In other words, a person could look great at 150 pounds, or a person could look terrible at that weight.

We could place potatoes or bricks or a person on a scale and read "150" on the dial. The scale tells us nothing about the quality or condition of weight. In other words, a person could look great at 150 pounds, or a person could look terrible at that weight. It is all determined by the composition of the body.

My preference for determining whether a person is overweight or obese is using a body-mass index that measures body fat percentage against the lean body or muscle weight. This method of determining body composition says much more than just weight does because it relates directly to health. (By the way, most YMCAs, health clubs and health fairs offer body fat testing.)

A female is considered clinically obese when her body fat is 30 percent or greater. A male is considered clinically obese when his body fat surpasses 25 percent. But the good news is that people can change their body composition through fitness programs, sports and physical activities that stimulate muscle growth. In other words, the amount they weigh can become composed of less fat and more muscle. And I believe that measuring gives a more accurate representation of health.

THE OBESITY-DISEASE CONNECTION

"MALIGNANT OBESITY" IS a term now used to define persons 60 percent above desirable weight; this corresponds to an absolute excess of 100 pounds. With this degree of obesity, there is a minimum doubling of all causes of morbidity and mortality.[12] Obese people who are diabetic or who have hypertension, heart disease or any other cardiovascular disease risk factor must reduce their weight. It is actually a matter of life or death.

Hypertension, or high blood pressure, is commonly associated with obesity. Overweight men and women from age twenty to their mid-forties are six times more likely to have hypertension than their same-aged peers of normal weight.[13] Of course, weight gain in young adults sets the stage for hypertension in later years.

Menopausal women whose excess fat has been localized in the upper torso (upper back, arms and stomach) have an increased risk of developing breast cancer. There are also higher rates of cancer of the uterus and ovaries among overweight women. Overweight men have a definite higher mortality rate for colorectal and prostate cancers.[14]

Being overweight places unnecessary trauma on the weight-bearing joints such as the knees. In middle-aged women, excess body weight is a major predictor of osteoarthritis of the knees. Every time overweight people reduce their body weight, they are increasing the longevity of their joints while improving their mobility to perform everyday tasks.

Weight and Your Health

The Obesity-Psychological Disorders Connection

BECAUSE OF THEIR excess weight and size, many obese individuals suffer from lower back and joint pain and inflammation as well as difficulty breathing. As a result, overweight people may struggle with issues of inadequacy or lowered self-worth related to the performance of normal day-to-day tasks at work, play or social interaction.

Additionally, people struggling with obesity may have felt discriminated against at one time or another, possibly in the work or academic setting. These psychological issues that are associated with poor body image are often a consequence of obesity.[15]

The Obesity-Diabetes Connection

NEARLY 80 PERCENT of patients with noninsulin-dependent diabetes mellitus are obese.[16] Many people with this type diabetes struggle with weight gain due to the lack of regular exercise. Since the body is not burning or metabolizing calories adequately, it stores them in the form of fat.

Excess body fat interferes with normal blood glucose levels. Because the body no longer handles insulin normally, the blood sugar or glucose builds up in the blood, and blood glucose levels increase. This generally is due to overeating or eating too much at one time. Regular exercise and weight loss will help normalize the blood sugar levels.

High-Glycemic Foods and Weight

OVER THE YEARS I have asked hundreds of clients and students to fill out a three-day dietary analysis of the foods and beverages they consume. From these, I noticed a common denominator: Most of them selected high-glycemic foods for over 80 percent of their diets!

High-glycemic foods are simple sugars or carbohydrates. They consist of single sugar molecules that convert to energy very quickly. When ingested, they provide immediate energy, which is great when a person is in need of raising glucose levels or requires an immediate lift for performing a task. But when too many high-glycemic foods are consumed, they can play havoc on our metabolism by slowing down the body's ability to burn calories and causing hypoglycemia, or low blood sugar.

Many people have been led to believe that a diet high in carbohydrates is healthy. But from all of my findings, both personally and professionally, I believe that most people are carrying too much body fat and are unhealthy because they are eating too many carbohydrates.

Typically, a glycemic index food chart lists the conversion rate of a food to energy, or how much the insulin level increases when that food is ingested. After food is ingested, the pancreas produces insulin. Insulin then does its job and transports truckloads of sugar over to the furnace or power plant in the cell to be burned. These power plants, called mitochondria, convert the sugar into usable energy. When too many simple sugars are ingested, the power plant becomes full. Then the overflow is stored in the liver and fat cells. This is not something you want if you are trying to lose weight! Too many simple sugars eaten day after day can also contribute to diabetes and other health problems.

Insulin's normal function is to escort glucose to your cells for energy conversion. However, a continual over-insulin response caused by the overconsumption of simple sugars (high-glycemic food) encourages fat storage. It causes low blood sugar, slows your metabolism, makes you tired and hungry, weakens your immune system and interferes with protein synthesis (your body's ability to build muscle or lean weight).

So, foods on the glycemic food chart are rated by number from 0 to 100, with 100 representing how high the insulin rises when straight glucose (sugar) is ingested. The foods with higher

HEALTH **FACT** BOX

GYLCEMIC INDEX
FOR SELECTED CARBOHYDRATES

The higher its glycemic index, the more significant effect a particular food will have on your blood sugar. Do your best to avoid foods with high numbers.

Glucose	100	Baked potatoes	95
White bread	95	Mashed potatoes	90
Honey	90	Carrots	85
Corn flakes, popcorn	85	Refined cereal	
Chocolate bar, candy bar	70	(with sugar)	70
Cookies	70	Boiled potatoes	70
White rice	70	Corn	70
Half bread (half white)			
half whole-grain)	65	Beets	65
Banana	60	Jam	55
White pasta	55	Whole-grain bread	50
Wheat rice	50	Peas	50
Complete cereal			
(no sugar)	50	Oat flakes	40
Fresh fruit juice			
(no sugar)	40	Rye bread	40
Wheat pasta	40	Dairy	35
Dry beans	30	Lentils	30
Garbanzo beans	30	Fresh fruit	30
Fruit marmalade			
(no sugar)	25	Fructose	20
Dark chocolate			
(more than 60% cocoa)	22	Soy	15
Green veggies, tomatoes, lemon, mushrooms			less than 5[17]

numbers are high-glycemic or quick-energy foods, such as candy bars, breads, juice, white bread, white rice, corn and sweeteners such as corn syrup, just to name a few.

If you are like most Americans today and get the majority of your calories from high-glycemic foods, then you are flirting with potential health and weight problems. To better control sugar cravings, stabilize blood sugar levels, promote weight loss and have more energy throughout each day, eat low-glycemic foods as your staples.

Use the lists in this chapter for reference when selecting low-glycemic foods and avoiding high-glycemic foods.

HEALTH FACT BOX

HIGH-GLYCEMIC FOODS

- Foods containing sugar, honey, molasses and corn syrup
- Fruits such as bananas, watermelon, pineapple and raisins
- Vegetables such as potatoes, corn, carrots, beets, turnips and parsnips
- Breads such as all-white breads, all-white flour products and corn breads
- Grains including rice, rice products, millet, corn and corn products
- Pasta, especially thick, large pasta shapes
- Cereals, including all cereals except those on the low-glycemic list below
- Snacks, especially potato chips, corn chips, popcorn, rice, cakes and pretzels
- Alcoholic beverages

HEALTH **FACT** BOX

Low-Glycemic Foods

- Foods sweetened with saccharin, aspartame or fructose
- All meats
- All dairy products (no sugars)
- Fruits, except the high-glycemic fruits listed
- Vegetables, except the high-glycemic vegetables listed
- Breads such as whole rye, pumpernickel and whole-wheat pita
- Grains, including barley, bulgar and kasha
- Pasta, such as thin strands, whole-wheat pasta and lean threads
- Cereals like Special K, All Bran, Fiber One and regular oatmeal
- Snacks, including nuts, olives, cheese and pita chips
- Red wine

Low-Glycemic Food Choices

IT WAS INTERESTING to observe the connection between the food choices my students recorded and the symptoms about which they complained: light-headedness, dizziness, brain fog, moderate to high obesity, sugar cravings and sometimes depression and irritability.

John attended my Fitness and Fellowship class, and one day he told all of us that after eating breakfast, he found it nearly impossible to keep his eyes open. By the time he drove to work he felt terrible. So I asked him what he was eating for breakfast. "Sometimes cereal and milk, or sometimes toast and coffee. But I always have a big glass of orange juice," he replied.

I made a couple of suggestions, one of which was to eliminate the orange juice. Only one week later he shared with the class that when he avoided the orange juice, his energy level stayed constant. Because he had been constantly ingesting a large amount of high-glycemic foods, he had become so intolerant to glucose that when he drank the high-glycemic juice, he would crash.

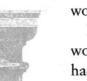

Before she could possibly expect to lose a pound, she had to learn how to put the sugar monster to sleep.

Laura was forty years old, a working mom and a housewife. She had been steadily gaining weight over the past few years and could now accurately be called overweight. Besides that, she had absolutely no energy. She felt particularly tired around ten o'clock in the morning and three o'clock in the afternoon. She said she couldn't lose weight. Laura also experienced depression and craved sweets. She definitely felt older than her age, she was always tired, and she was borderline diabetic.

Laura's dietary analysis showed that she skipped breakfast, snacked on candy bars and cookies, drank up to ten cans of soda a day and ate her largest meal at night.

Unbeknownst to her, she revealed herself to be an expert at feeding the sugar monster that produced all the symptoms of her high-glycemic diet. Before she could possibly expect to lose a pound, she had to learn how to put the sugar monster to sleep.

The key factor in doing this is remembering that every time we ingest fuel (food), a biochemical reaction takes place. In her case, the high-glycemic diet was inducing a hypoglycemic reaction. As she continued eating these types of foods day in and day out, her pancreas constantly was being overstimulated. Consequently, she was creating too high an insulin response too often.

This caused her metabolism to slow down, which contributed to her weight gain. The overstimulated insulin response caused by the simple sugars she ate regularly stole sugar from her blood, causing her to feel tired every day. And because of her lack of physical activity, those simple sugars or carbohydrates she was eating converted into stored fat.

You can see how frustrating it was for her. She was trying to lose weight, have more energy and feel alive. But she was doing all the wrong things—things that prohibited weight loss and made her feel tired and depressed.

Laura came to our group fitness class, which consisted of three forty-five-minute exercise sessions a week. I outlined some basic dietary guidelines for her to follow that would serve as a starting point: Eat low-glycemic foods that were compatible with her blood type; add protein to her meals; and have protein shakes between meals. I also suggested that she take a few dietary supplements on a regular basis. I knew if she would follow these few suggestions as best as she could, there was hope.

Laura herself took the biggest step of all—getting off the couch.

Two weeks later, when she entered the fitness class, she had a new glow to her skin and a sparkle in her eyes. She really looked fresh, healthier and alive. Laura told me that her energy remained level throughout the day and that she felt better than she had in years. Now she had a clear mind and did not crave sugar.

If you want to gain better control of your sweet tooth, overcome those feelings of depression and sluggishness and avoid potential serious health problems, then eliminate or minimize your simple sugars and replace them with low-glycemic or complex

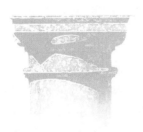

carbohydrates. These are the foods numbered from 0 to 50 on the glycemic index chart. Low-glycemic foods contain multichain molecules that burn more slowly, like a time-released food. They do not give a quick spike of insulin and immediate energy, but rather they promote an

By eating lower glycemic foods, you can put the sugar monster to sleep forever.

even insulin response and convert to energy over a longer period of time.

For example, switching from a simple sugar to a complex carbohydrate could mean going from white rice to brown rice. You don't have to go without—just make some switches that will give you a steady energy level, less spiking in your insulin response and more control over craving sweets. Plus, they will enhance your metabolic process.

Over the next few weeks Laura dropped pounds and inches—something she wasn't able to do before. Now her body was beginning to function the way it was originally designed to function. It could perform optimally for her at last.

Once we get the machine in good operating order, the rest is a "piece of cake"!

Speaking of cake, there is nothing wrong with having those occasional goodies. The problems begin when they are the rule instead of the exception. If you walk by a dessert tray and feel like having something sweet, then go for it. But if you walk by that tray and it grabs you like a vice grip and says, "Eat me or else," then the sugar monster is still wide awake in you. By eating lower glycemic foods, you can put the sugar monster to sleep forever.

PROTEIN—STIMULUS FOR WEIGHT LOSS

JUST AS CARBOHYDRATES stimulate an insulin response, protein stimulates another hormone named glucagon. Functioning opposite of insulin, glucagon encourages the body to burn fats, stabilizes the blood sugar, strengthens the immune system, suppresses the appetite and supports protein synthesis. Glucagon, when stimulated by protein, will cause the body to burn fat more readily, reduce hunger and cravings for sweets and protect the immune system. It is responsible for aiding the body to maintain lean weight.

So, if you are on a high-carbohydrate and low-protein diet, you can see why it will be virtually impossible to lose weight or fat. Your body needs adequate amounts of protein daily. As a rule, you should ingest 1 gram of protein for every 2.2 pounds of body weight. If you exercise regularly and are very physically active, then I would recommend 1 to 1.5 or more grams of protein per 2.2 pounds of body weight.

To stimulate weight loss, make sure your meals and snacks favor protein over carbohydrates. Eating a meal that has more protein calories than carbohydrate calories is considered to be an anabolic meal. Creating anabolic momentum will cause your body to burn fat for energy, thereby stabilizing blood sugar levels and supplying the muscle tissues with the nutrition needed for repair and building.

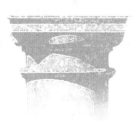

Should you choose to eat from the glycemic index and the protein chart, make sure your food selections are compatible to your blood

To stimulate weight loss, make sure your meals and snacks favor protein over carbohydrates.

type (we'll get to that next). When followed correctly, this will not feel like going on a diet. Instead, it will allow your body to function properly and will improve your digestive and immune system.

HEALTH FACT BOX

PROTEIN CHOICES

Here are some protein-rich foods that you can choose from to go with your meals or snacks. All meats should be lean. Do not eat deli meats.

- Turkey and chicken
- Eggs, egg whites or egg substitute
- Low-fat cottage cheese
- Low-fat yogurt
- Tofu
- Fish—broiled or baked
- Red meat
- Low-fat cheese
- Nuts
- Protein shakes

STAYING HYDRATED

DRINKING ENOUGH WATER is critical to staying well. Try drinking a glass of water every hour. Spike it with lemon or lime, or drink sparkling water if that's what it takes to get you to do it. To find out the amount of water you should drink daily, convert one-half of your body weight to ounces. That's how many ounces of water you should drink daily. For example, if you weigh 150 pounds, you need 75 ounces of water a day.

Avoid or minimize sodas and fruit drinks, and avoid fruit juices made from concentrates. Herbal teas, particularly green tea, are better choices than coffee. Also, drinks with caffeine will contribute to dehydration, so avoid those as well.

Weight and Your Health

EATING FOR WEIGHT
MANAGEMENT

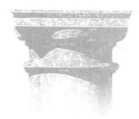

THE INCLINATION TO become fat or overweight is induced by lifestyles that lack physical activities and are full of poor food selections, including an abundance of processed and fast foods. We'll talk about the role of exercise and being active in Pillar V. And Pillar II will help you make good food choices and set you free from dieting forever.

Food nourishes our bodies, not our minds or emotions. There is nothing on your plate that can meet your emotional needs.

But for now, remember these three guidelines:

1. Eat when you are hungry.
2. Eat until you are satisfied (not stuffed).
3. Put the brakes on and stop eating if you are full.

Food nourishes our bodies, not our minds or emotions. There is nothing on your plate that can meet your emotional needs.

Regardless of how you feel, your emotions should not be allowed to cross over to your plate of food. Remember, a classic example of an emotional eater is a person who eats when he or she is not hungry. We do damage to our bodies, our minds and our relationships with others by not having the proper boundaries in place.

If you are anxious or tense, go for a walk or have a workout. If you are depressed or feeling unneeded, call a friend who will make you laugh. When you feel stressed, pray and do relaxation exercises (see Pillar VI). When you are angry, forgive. When you are sad, hug someone. When you are tired, go to sleep. Whatever emotional state you are in, remember that there is Someone who loves you unconditionally—God!

Seven Pillars of Health

Let me encourage you: Once you learn some of the basics of weight management included here in Pillar I and in the next Pillar on Diet, you will find weight management one of the easiest of the Seven Pillars of Health to keep intact.

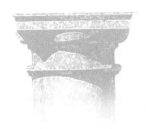

I'm sure you can now see the value in keeping this Pillar of Weight Management from cracking. No doubt you have already created fitness and nutrition goals you want to reach—plans for your future and the future of your loved ones. Write them down now as you get ready to take action on the Pillar of Weight Management.

You are not what you think you are. What you think, you are!

Imagine that you and I could sit down for an hour or two and plan out what could be done to strengthen your Pillar of Weight Management. Would you take all the information and guidelines and make them a part of your lifestyle, or would they just become dust collectors?

The success of our plan for you would boil down to your integrity. Whether you accomplish what you set out to do or not will be determined by the lifestyle you choose to live.

Attitudes determine actions. You are not what you think you are. What you think, you are!

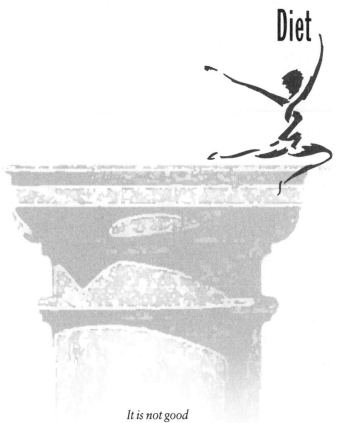

Diet

2

It is not good
to eat too *much honey.*
—PROVERBS 25:27

PILLAR TWO

4

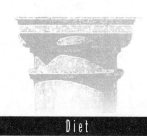

THE DESPAIR
OF DIETING

Oh, no!" came the scream from the warm-up room.

My student and I looked at each other in surprise. Though we were training a room away, we still heard the shriek. Should we go to see what happened? Before we could decide, we heard the stationary bike going furiously. That sound brought knowing smiles to our lips as we realized what the scream of despair was all about.

In the late eighties, I owned and operated several personal training studios in which I offered private one-on-one personal training as well as nutritional counseling. As students arrived, they went directly to the warm-up room to spend the first fifteen minutes biking in preparation for the thirty-minute circuit training workout we would do together.

Both at the request of my students and for the purpose of calculating body fat percentages, I put scales in the warm-up rooms. Most students jumped on a scale as soon as they entered to see if they were winning the battle—or to see how badly they were losing it! For some reason, the scales were most prevalently used on Monday mornings. On this particular Monday morning, the

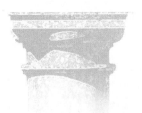

Sadly, most people would rather wallow in the familiar ignorance of going on a diet than be willing to accept unfamiliar truths.

number on the scale evoked a scream from Mary.

As soon I finished training my student, Mary came in to start her workout. I politely didn't mention her scream. However, as we started training, I asked how her weekend had gone. That was all it took for the tears to start flowing.

Overwhelmed by guilt, Mary began confessing all her dietary sins to me. She told me how badly she had done over the weekend and how guilty she felt for eating foods she was not allowed to eat. She wistfully told me how she had been doing good for a while on her diet, but then she went off it and began to binge. After giving me a rundown of the foods she ate, she was nearly exhausted. I had to stop her in the middle of the workout to get her calmed down.

I wasn't completely shocked by her state of mind because the scream from the warm-up room was all too familiar. But being a former 305-pound dough boy myself, my heart went out to her. I felt her struggle to beat this weight problem, and I felt her pain of defeat.

So I gently reminded her of my philosophy—one that I believed would break this cycle of guilt and pain. "Mary, do you remember that I didn't teach you to diet to lose weight? So how could you have 'gone off' your diet?"

"I read about a diet in a ladies' magazine," she blurted out. "It guaranteed to drop several pounds in just a few days. So I started it, but I couldn't stay on it."

I knew her intentions were good, and she was determined to succeed. But she, like so many others who are victimized by their own desperation, easily fell prey to information that offered a quick remedy to her problem. In Mary's case, her desperation put her in touch with the wrong approach to getting her weight under control—one that would not bring ultimate success.

It's sometimes frightening to think how many people live in fear and trembling when it comes to weight and diet. The emotional stress levels that people reach when they go on a diet are totally unnecessary.

The scale means little when it comes to monitoring the success of eating to lose weight. Weight management is multidimensional, and eating is just one aspect of it. Sadly, most people would rather wallow in the familiar ignorance of going on a diet than be willing to accept unfamiliar truths. For some, it must feel safer to stay within their comfort zones, to keep following the same ways that have over and over proved to be unsuccessful, somehow retaining the hope that one day success will come. That is a true way of going insane.

A Trip to Diet Island

Let me take you on a journey to Diet Island, though I never expect you to go on this journey again! For now, just sit back and enjoy the cruise as this ship takes you away to an island where "going on a diet" is king.

The cruise begins on Friday night. As you step onto the cruise ship, you notice how well-appointed it is. You are sure you are going to enjoy the ride to Diet Island. Somehow the atmosphere seems to promise that you will finally be happy, that soon you will feel good enough about yourself to lie on a white sand beach in a bikini.

Your thoughts are interrupted by the dinner bell, and boy, is dinner scrumptious! You don't want to miss a thing, so later you have the midnight snack even though you aren't hungry.

On Saturday morning you eat a full breakfast and enjoy walking on the deck. Then comes the barbecue on the promenade. Someone reminds you to stay up for the midnight dessert buffet; you don't have to be told twice.

Seven Pillars of Health

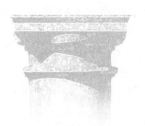

On Sunday you skip breakfast and sleep in. The Sunday brunch, though, is worth getting up for. Then, after a lazy afternoon of lounging on the deck, you decide just to have dessert for dinner. But that doesn't really fill you up, so you go to the late-night buffet as well.

That's OK, you think. I can handle this diet for a while. It's only for a few weeks. Then I'll have the rest of my life to enjoy food again. The reward will be worth it.

As you enjoy the ride, your mind wanders back. You heard about your destination, Diet Island, from someone, somewhere, who told you how someone she knew went to this island and lost fifteen pounds in just ten days. You can't wait to have results like that. It will be worth the sacrifice.

Early Monday morning the island comes into view. You don't see any of the lush tropical vegetation and pristine beaches you expected. In fact, it looks like it's a desert island... mostly stretches of dry, hot sand with just a few scrawny weeds here and there. *That's OK,* you tell yourself. *I've finally made a commitment that once and for all I will be free of fat—no matter what.*

Of course, you will need to be taught how to go on a diet, so you are met at the dock by your new teacher. Your teacher's name is Mr. Diet. Later, you find out from another visitor that his first name is Going Ona, but he doesn't like people to know that.

After a quick drink of water (you wish it had been a cold soda), you are led to the introductory session. You find Mr. Diet inflexible and unforgiving. He reveals that all the information you will receive there is only good for the time that you are on the island. It's no good once you go back home.

That's OK, you tell yourself. *I'll have everything I need by the time I leave here.*

The Despair of Dieting

At this point Mr. Diet takes total control of your life. He lists the rules of behavior, which must be followed to the tee. Severe penalties await you if you violate any of them. Plus, there is no leaving the island to have fun. You are not allowed to enjoy life or enjoy any food as long as you are on this island. And that is the way it will be for the duration.

That's OK, you think. *I can handle this diet for a while. It's only for a few weeks. Then I'll have the rest of my life to enjoy food again. The reward will be worth it.*

"It's uncertain how long you will spend on this island. It could be two or three weeks, a few months—or even the rest of your life. It all depends on your will power," the teacher sternly informs you. A chill runs down your spine, but you ignore it.

After a full 12-ounce glass of water and two carrots, your classroom instruction begins. You learn that eating is basically a system of punishment and reward. Your ability to muster up enough will power to stay on your diet will determine how many rewards you receive. So you must work diligently at using your will power.

To ensure your success, you are constantly reminded and warned of the devastation that you will cause to yourself if for some reason you should go "off" your diet. Going off your diet is unacceptable, and there will be severe penalties applied, including guilt, frustration and a sense of failure.

First, you must avoid any and all foods that you like or that taste good. "Nutritious can never be delicious." You have to memorize that mantra. You must learn how to sacrifice, to go without and to accept deprivation as a virtue.

Second, you must learn to eat very few calories because calories are your worst enemy. You will become so familiar with your enemy on this island that you will know the exact number in their army no matter in which food they come hidden. If you lose count, you are told, they will overtake and conquer you.

Hand in hand with counting calories is starvation. You must learn the art of starvation and deprivation so that you don't go off your diet and commit the one cardinal dietary sin—the binge. This sin will cause such defeat that the teacher rails against it for a long time.

That's OK, you tell yourself. *None of this really matters because I've been around long enough to know that dieting is the only way to lose weight.* So you're pumped and ready to suck it up. What's the big deal about going on a diet anyway? You can do it.

After reviewing your diet plan, Mr. Diet gives you the main tool for determining your success—a bathroom scale. Yes, now you are ready to begin the regimen.

The first thing that you do the next morning and every morning that follows is weigh yourself. For the first two weeks you see the scale reading less and less each day, and you are thrilled. You are beginning to feel good about yourself. In fact, you can almost look into the mirror without cringing. *Bikini, here I come!* You feel very positive that this time the diet is not going to let you down. It's actually working. You've cut back on your calories, you've learned how to starve and deprive yourself, you're going without—and you're dropping weight.

Then, after the first three weeks, something just isn't right. You feel tired all the time, and you're not as chipper as you were before. Plus, your weight has quit going down. It isn't going up, but it isn't going down, either. *How can this be happening?* You're doing everything Mr. Diet told you to do.

In a state of panic you decide to make some changes to your diet—covertly, of course. You cut back on calories because they are the enemy. That should fix the problem.

The next day and the next you go back to the scale for the reward, but no weight has been lost. *What's wrong?* Now you feel a sense of urgency—almost panic. Every morning, noon and night you weigh yourself to look for your reward. All this sacrificing to

The Despair of Dieting

no avail? Impossible! But the scale is not changing. You have stopped dropping weight.

Not only has the scale become unfriendly, but you feel worse than ever. You're terribly grumpy and irritable, and nobody can come near you. You feel less and less able to cope with the lack of nutrition, and what's worse—you're hungry. You are so hungry that you can't think of anything but all those good-tasting foods that your teacher said you must sacrifice. The cravings are driving you crazy.

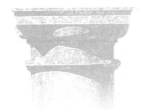

You recognize these horrifying warning signs—the signs that signal the attack of the dietary cardinal sin. But you can no longer help yourself. You fought it the best you could, and your will power is gone. Your determination and desire have been

If you have dieted before, then you have probably experienced the drudgery of a weight-loss diet—and how unrealistic sticking to it can be.

overcome by weakness and hunger. All your effort and sacrifice are a thing of the past. You are out of control and ready to binge.

You stow away on the next ship that leaves—a cargo ship that is bringing vegetables to the island—and as soon as you arrive on land, you race to the first fast-food place, ice cream stand or doughnut shop that you spot. You are completely out of control, and the cravings for sugar are so strong that you would kill for something sweet.

The cruise is over, the island adventure is shot and your diet has turned out to be your enemy. Once again, you've become frustrated, discouraged and more depressed than before you went to the island. Over the next couple of weeks, the weight comes back on, and you wonder how many extra pounds it will take before you drum up enough will power to return to Diet Island again.

Seven Pillars of Health

IF YOU HAVE been around the last twenty years or so, I'm certain you have visited Diet Island once or twice. That's because dieting has become a way of life for many. If you have been to Diet Island, there is a good chance that you are included somewhere in the following statistics:[1]

1. More than one in five children ages 6 through 17 are overweight.

2. Thirty-two million American women between the ages of 20 and 74 are overweight.

3. Americans spend nearly $10 billion per year on diet aids.

4. In 1998, 27 percent of U.S. adults were currently dieting.

5. Only 5 percent of all dieters will have maintained their weight.

The quick-fix approach to losing weight will not bring you success, and its effects on your health and appearance will not be positive. If you have dieted before, then you have probably experienced the drudgery of a weight-loss diet—and how unrealistic sticking to it can be.

But we'll discover that learning the difference between going on a weight-loss diet and eating a healthy, well-balanced diet is the first step toward long-term success.

It's great to be known as a person who has a lot of will power. But will power is not the key that unlocks the door to dietary freedom. Neither is starvation or deprivation. On the contrary, those dietary approaches are outdated, physiologically inaccurate and should never be a part of your life again. They are directly responsible for

The Despair of Dieting

keeping your body fat. Your dieting efforts have proven one basic truth: Weight loss from dieting is temporary at best and makes your body fatter than when you started the diet.

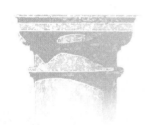

When doing seminars on weight management and diets, my favorite question for my audience is, "How many of you have ever gone on a diet to lose weight?" Usually, about 85 percent of the people

Weight loss from dieting is temporary at best and makes your body fatter than when you started the diet.

raise their hands. Then I ask the next question, "How many of you lost weight?" About 60 percent respond positively. Then I asked the big one, "How many of you who lost weight on your weight-loss diets have gained it back again?" Just about 90 percent of them indicate they have.

What does that say about dieting? Did they fail, did the diet plan fail, or is the idea of dieting a failure?

My goal is to set you free from the bondage of dieting by raising your awareness of what dieting is and is not. You will learn that you are free to enjoy food without the sense of guilt that so often accompanies the dieting mentality. You will be set free from the yo-yo syndrome and the fear of going off your diet.

That's why this information will not lead you to go on a diet. You will experience dietary freedom for the first time in your life, while at the same time maintaining a healthy body weight and a potentially disease-free life that is full of energy. The frustration, self-inflicted stress and the tremendous sense of failure associated with dieting to lose weight will become a thing of the past. You will embark on a brand-new approach to eating that will literally set you free from the bondage of dieting.

49

5

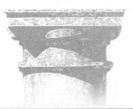

THE BLOOD TYPE
CONNECTION
TO DIET

This Diet Pillar of Health is the one most likely to play havoc with the health of your superstructure. Its potential for developing cracks is extremely high, because this Pillar seems to be the most neglected, misinterpreted, misunderstood and most abused Pillar of all. So in order to understand what *diet* means, let's look at a simple dictionary definition.

Webster's has several definitions for the word *diet*. A diet can be "to cause to eat and drink sparingly or according to prescribed rules." It can also mean, "Food and drink that are regularly provided and consumed." Did you notice that there is a difference between the idea of *going on a diet* and the noun *diet?* One is a set of rules, and the other is the food you regularly eat. Your knowledge of this distinction will make all the difference in the world to your success. One will put you in prison, and the other will set you free.

PASSING OUT AND ANSWERED PRAYER

FOR THE GREATER part of my life I have been a fairly healthy person. But sometime in 1986 I felt my health going downhill. I was losing the ability to function normally on a day-to-day basis. I wasn't sure what was wrong, but it was like having to endure a nightmare during the day.

Every day around ten in the morning and three in the afternoon I would crash. I could actually roll over and fall asleep in the middle of a training session, business meeting or while driving my car. I realized that I had been experiencing these symptoms for about five years, but they were getting worse.

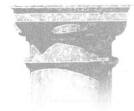

Immediately after I ate I had tons of energy and felt great, but within an hour or so, my energy dropped like a roller coaster.

At the time I was buried in my personal training business, which required long days, most of my energy and time, plus all the stress I could handle. For lunch I would usually go out for some Chinese food, such as my favorite, chicken-fried rice. Then I would go back to the studio.

Immediately after I ate I had tons of energy and felt great, but within an hour or so, my energy dropped like a roller coaster. I would be in the middle of a training session with a client, and yet I could hardly keep my eyes open. Not only was I tired and sleepy, but many times I would feel anxious, light-headed and lethargic. Mentally I was in a brain fog. I even had the feeling of being depressed—without an apparent reason.

One evening in 1986 Lori and I were out for a drive. We had splurged on a couple of candy bars—you know, the all-American health snack. I needed to gas up the car, so I pulled into the service station. However, when I tried to get out to pump the gas, I just couldn't because I felt so weak. I had to ask Lori to pump the gas because I could not keep my eyes open a moment longer. It was just as if I were poisoned. Graciously she agreed, and by the time she got back into the car, I had passed out at the wheel.

That incident led me to see a doctor for some tests, including a glucose test, which came out positive. I was suffering from hypoglycemia, or low blood sugar. I was given a few books on the topic to read as well as a list of foods—forbidden and permissible. Can you imagine having to live that way? That just wasn't acceptable to me. I promised myself that I would find another way to correct this debilitating condition.

In the meantime, I followed the list, but eating the prescribed foods didn't give me much relief. The physician advised me to incorporate some milk for a protein source, which would slow down the insulin response. Also, I was put on wheat bread instead of white. However, adding those two foods did not help.

Hypoglycemia, or low blood sugar, occurs when blood levels of glucose (a form of sugar that is the body's main fuel) drop too low to fuel the body's activity. The symptoms of hypoglycemia can include drowsiness, weakness, dizziness, hunger and confusion. At times headache, irritability, trembling, rapid heart beat, sweating and a cold, clammy feeling may also be symptoms. In severe cases a person may lose consciousness or even lapse into a coma.[1]

I struggled for another ten years, sometimes getting a handle on my health, but mostly just trying to survive. Keep in mind, this whole time I was in the fitness business! It was so overwhelming that I used to ask the Lord to show me what I could do about getting healed. If I had to live like that for the rest of my life, I would dread living. How horrible life can be when your health is upside down!

My condition prompted me to research more studies and to experiment personally. First, I learned about high-glycemic foods, and I incorporated the use of the glycemic index for making food selections because I thought it would help control my hypo-glycemia. I did start to feel a little change for the better. My blood sugar seemed to level out more often than before, but I still struggled and still crashed every day.

IT ALL MADE SENSE

FINALLY IN THE summer of 1997, I found the answer to my prayers. I had been reading information about the link that exists between people's blood type and what they should eat. Since I had been involved in the health and fitness industry for over thirty years, I was quite familiar with all the dieting fads that came in vogue for a while and then fizzled out like a Fourth of July firecracker. But this was different. It made all the sense in the world to me.

I devoured the studies and the research that showed the link between blood type, diet and disease. What impressed me the most was the concept that certain foods were better for one person than others because of that person's individual cellular profile. This was not the same old idea that one diet fits all.

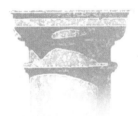

This was not the same old idea that one diet fits all.

Since most weight-loss diets are designed for anyone and everyone, they do not take into consideration the genetic makeup of each individual. Consequently, they lack accuracy. One-diet-for-everyone is common protocol for dieticians, nutritionists and the average healthcare practitioner. The fact that special diets are given to heart patients, diabetics and people with various other illnesses and diseases shows some improvement in this arena. But these professionals still haven't seemed to make the connection that one diet doesn't suit every person. A diet plan that suggests that it will work for everyone is ludicrous and old school—and should send up a red flag for you.

Seven Pillars of Health

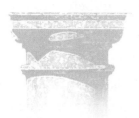

I decided to give this new way of eating a try. When I learned which foods were most compatible for my blood type and which were actually toxic for my blood type, I made the appropriate dietary adjustments.

When I did, something happened to me that I hadn't experienced in about fifteen years. Besides immediately losing body fat and muscularizing my physique even more, I no longer experienced the gas and bloating that used to be normal after eating a meal. Plus, I had constant energy throughout the entire day. The brain fog was gone. Finally, no more crashing! After all the months and years I spent wasting my time with diet plans, it only took about five days of eating correctly for my blood type for my blood sugar to stabilize. Thank God I have kept a stable blood sugar level ever since.

After all the months and years I spent wasting my time with diet plans, it only took about five days of eating correctly for my blood type for my blood sugar to stabilize.

Learning about the association between blood types and diet, then personally experiencing the results for myself, has made me a firm believer that this approach to healthy eating is the most accurate way of making proper food choices. Eating correctly for your blood type will give new hope to anyone who is interested in a healthier, more energetic and disease-free life.

THE EXCITING RESULTS

MY BLOOD TYPE is O, and therefore I am genetically designed to be a red meat eater. That might sound alarming to you because it goes against the current thinking that red meat is an unhealthy source of protein. But that is not true for blood type O people.

Before I started eating this way, I had red meat maybe once a month. But as soon as I understood that people with O blood type are compatible for digesting, assimilating and utilizing red meat, I decided to try eating it more often. I decided that if I were going to benefit from this relatively new concept, I would have to give a 100 percent effort. So I did.

For the first six months I ate approximately one to two pounds of red meat daily as my primary source of protein. I also ate plenty of veggies and fruits that were compatible for my type. Additionally, I avoided the foods that were not compatible, at least the best I could. Plus, I avoided so-called junk foods 95 percent of the time.

Here is an idea of what I ate. For breakfast, I had one to three eggs and a beef pattie or one to two slices of Ezekiel bread (made from sprouted grain) toasted with butter. If I ate only toast, I would put almond spread and natural-juice black cherry jam on it, then have a blood type-compatible chocolate protein drink and sparkling water. Of course, I took supplements every morning.

Midmorning I usually had some walnuts and pitted prunes. Sometimes I would enjoy a chocolate protein shake instead. For lunch I ate a chicken Caesar salad, liver and broccoli or perhaps an 8-ounce petite sirloin with a sweet potato and a Caesar salad. My midafternoon snack was the same as my morning snack. My evening meal would be similar to my lunch. Usually I ate green veggies with all meals. With every meal I drank sparkling water. If I was hungry, I'd drink a chocolate protein shake in the evening.

At the end of those six months I thought it wise to get some blood work done and see how my body was reacting to this new way of eating. The outside of my house was looking good, but I needed a look at the inside.

When I got my blood work results back I was elated. They were better than I had hoped. My total cholesterol was down from 180 to 150, my HDL (good cholesterol) read 49, my LDL (bad cholesterol) read 87, and my triglycerides were 68. What did all that mean?

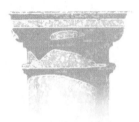

When I got my blood work results back I was elated. They were better than I had hoped.

Simply put, after adding red meat to my diet as a staple protein source for six months and avoiding the foods incompatible to my blood type, my blood work showed me that my blood lipids, or fats, were in the low normal ranges. That meant that (contrary to current opinion) my intake of animal protein *did not* induce elevated cholesterol levels. In fact, it contributed to lowering them.

Astonishing? Not for a type O! Does that mean everyone can eat red meat as their primary source of protein? No, but a blood type O can.

As you can imagine, I became totally convinced that this approach to eating was not only the most logical way of eating, but also the most scientifically sound because it was genetically based.

And the best part was, I felt set free. I said good-bye to dieting and hello to instinctive eating.

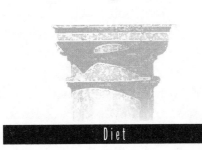

6

INSTINCTIVE EATING

W hen we eat, biochemical reactions to the foods we ingest occur within our bodies. These specific reactions are a part of our natural biological design. The way each of our bodies reacts to particular foods is the most accurate monitoring tool we can use for losing weight, improving energy, stabilizing blood sugar, controlling cholesterol levels and defeating a host of other health-related disorders that interfere with our ability to lead healthy and energetic lives. Learning to listen to and obey our bodies is called *instinctive eating.*

If we were like the animals, we probably would not have health-related problems associated with the foods we eat. No one has to tell a lion to eat red meat, and you would never catch one climbing a banana tree for bananas. Why? Because animals instinctively know what to eat. Not so for us humans. Our food choices are usually prompted by social gatherings, traditions, religious rules, emotions, church fellowships and advertisements, to name a few. In general, you name it, and we'll eat it.

We have gotten so out of touch with eating properly that we have accepted a reward and punishment system for selecting our nutrition. We base our food selections on our emotional state. Healthy foods are often a punishment for having overeaten. But junk foods are emotional rewards.

The biochemical reactions induced by the foods you eat are directly connected to *your* own genetic predisposition or makeup. Becoming aware of how your body reacts to food is the first place to start. You have to teach yourself to listen to your body. Let your body, not a diet plan, be your teacher.

LEARNING TO
LISTEN TO OUR BODIES

I SUPPOSE IF our Creator had designed us so that every time we ingested something that was not compatible with us we would get violently ill, then we might become instinctive eaters in a hurry. Our bodies do have specific responses to different foods, though they are not usually violent. But most of us are not listening to the more subtle ways our bodies react.

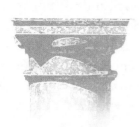

When I learned to avoid the foods that were not compatible with my blood type, not only did the heartburn disappear, but so did the gas, the bloating and the weight.

The beauty of eating correctly for blood type is that the biochemical reactions and responses to the foods we ingest become our dietary teacher. We just have to pay attention to them. This approach to eating allows our bodies to do the talking, and I'll show you how to listen.

Let me use myself as an example. Being Italian, I ate pasta, tomato sauce and black pepper four to five times a week. Following the meal came heartburn, gas and bloating. Now if that isn't a negative reaction, I don't what is.

Instinctive Eating

But I wasn't paying attention to my body's responses, and I wasn't aware of the association of food with blood type. So I took a spoonful of some pink stuff to put out the fire in my chest.

Until I learned to listen to my body, I didn't make the connection between my body's reaction and my health. Biochemical reactions such as these prove beyond a shadow of a doubt that everyone is not the same, and all diets should not be either. Rather, reactions like these should promote instinctive eating—the most natural and individualized way to make food selections.

First, we eat for the wrong reasons. Then, because we don't listen to our bodies, we find ourselves in deep trouble. Remember, if we violate the physical laws long enough, we are going to pay.

When I learned to avoid the foods that were not compatible with my blood type, not only did the heartburn disappear, but so did the gas, the bloating and the weight.

Keep in mind that not all foods will cause a negative reaction that is crippling or disruptive. Some incompatible foods contribute to illness and disease without notice. But many incompatible foods will give you signs, so watch for these after eating: weakness, gas, bloating, diarrhea, stomachache or acid reflux.

The more you adhere to eating the correct foods for your blood type, the more dramatic your body's negative responses will become when you eat the wrong ones.

Foods incompatible to your blood type are not just the foods you and I would consider junk food—potato chips, candy and dessert. In many cases foods you love to eat and think are healthy may be incompatible. Some of these can contribute to elevated cholesterol, while others slow your metabolism and interfere with your body's ability to lose weight. Incompatible foods can cause low blood sugar and hypoglycemia as well as gas, bloating, indigestion and irritable bowel syndrome.

HEALTH FACT BOX

Remember that the foods that are incompatible for myself and other blood type O people may not be incompatible for a blood type B person. As I mentioned earlier, red meat is desirable meat for my blood type. However, it would be very unwise for me to sit down to a big dinner of catfish—something a blood type B person could eat without experiencing the problems I would have.

In much the same way, a blood type AB individual may order a large fruit salad made with cantaloupe and honeydew melons served with cubes of cheddar cheese. But that person's blood type A lunch partner would need to avoid those melons and cheese, and perhaps choose some fat-free corn chips served with guacamole—something his blood type AB lunch partner must avoid.

When you eat compatible foods and avoid the incompatible ones, your body actually undergoes a detoxification. Your bodily systems—the digestive system, colon, kidneys, liver and the immune system—begin to operate as they were designed to. After the body adjusts to the compatible foods, an improvement in bodily function and performance follows. With a smoother operating machine, the body can rid itself of the toxins that are stored in the fat cells.

Compatible and incompatible foods also affect weight loss. Say, for example, a blood type O person needs to lose some excess fat,

HEALTH FACT BOX

Let's take a look at what our four lunch partners may choose for lunch—assuming they are each eating foods that are compatible for them.

Our blood type A person might decide to eat a bowl of lentil soup with a romaine lettuce salad with carrots, onions, artichoke, alfalfa sprouts and grilled tofu. Blood type AB might order red beans and rice with a side of broccoli. Blood type B may have 6 ounces of sliced turkey breast on a croissant with a side of cole slaw. My blood type O friend would probably stick with a small, broiled T-bone steak served with a side of green beans. And each person would leave the lunch table feeling great!

but she decides to eat foods that are made from wheat, thinking that wheat products are healthy. Well, it won't work for her. For a blood type O, wheat products actually slow down the body's metabolic process and make it difficult to lose weight. The digestive system cannot function properly until the compatible foods for the blood type are ingested.

The beauty of eating for your blood type if you are concerned about your weight is that losing fat is a natural by-product. Because you eliminate the incompatible foods from your diet, the toxins once stored in the fat cells will be eliminated. This causes the fat cells to shrink.

We may think that just junk foods are detrimental to our health. But in fact, it may be common, everyday foods that are interfering with your particular biochemistry.

The way your body responds to the foods you eat, whether it be negatively or positively, should be your monitoring tool to determine what food selections you should make. If you are on a special diet, or if you are eating according to another plan, such as the government's food pyramid, then choose foods compatible to your blood type from among those on your plan.

HEALTH FACT BOX

Here are a few foods that promote weight gain or loss for each blood type.

Blood Type A
- Weight gain: red meat and lima beans
- Weight loss: vegetables and soy products

Blood Type B
- Weight gain: peanuts and wheat
- Weight loss: meats and vegetables

Blood Type AB
- Weight gain: red meat and lima beans
- Weight loss: some red meat, soy products and vegetables

Blood Type O
- Weight gain: wheat products and cauliflower
- Weight loss: red meat and broccoli

Instinctive Eating

AFTER MY OWN success, I became compelled to share this revolutionary way of eating with everyone I came across. I changed the nutritional programs for my clients from what I thought had been healthy eating guidelines to the guidelines related to eating for their blood type.

Some of my clients immediately started losing weight. None of them ever felt hungry—in fact, they would comment on how satisfied they were. Some reported that their energy levels stayed constant, so I knew their blood sugar had stabilized.

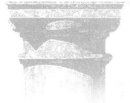

The beauty of eating for your blood type if you are concerned about your weight is that losing fat is a natural by-product. Because you eliminate the incompatible foods from your diet, the toxins once stored in the fat cells will be eliminated. This causes the fat cells to shrink.

As co-author of *The Answer Is in Your Bloodtype,* I receive feedback from people all over the country who are eating foods compatible to their blood type—and they all tell the same thing. As they are diligent not to eat the incompatible foods, they feel better, have more energy and lose body fat. That's because their bodies are getting a spring cleaning. The digestive system functions better, the blood sugar is more stable and the people perform at a higher level of maximized health.

Carol

Carol, a woman who flew with commercial airlines, came to our class interested but skeptical of this approach to eating because she had never heard it before. However, she decided to remove just one of the foods from a food group that was considered incompatible for her blood type. In her case, as a blood type O, she avoided pasta.

At that time her cholesterol was 230, and Carol admitted it was always high. One month after making only this one dietary change, her new cholesterol reading was 213. Needless to say she was ecstatic.

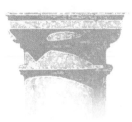

Most who follow the blood type approach to eating say they feel free to eat, generally are not hungry and have lost their cravings for sweets.

Now more convinced than ever, she removed more incompatible foods from her diet. After another month she had blood work done again. Her cholesterol level had dropped to 160. Her body had automatically started repairing and improving her bodily functions and systemic processes.

Carol's outer temple was also improving. In three months she dropped several dress sizes and shed approximately eighteen pounds. Today she is a believer—as is everybody else who learns to eat what they are and not go on a diet!

Gennie

I remember another student, Gennie, who was a dietaholic and hated the thought of exercise. In fact, she was the spitting image of the deconditioned, aging baby boomer of the new millennium. At forty-seven years of age she needed a major overhaul—and badly. We encouraged her to join the class and just give it her best shot.

Gennie had tried Jenny Craig, Weigh Down and everything else. She wasn't quite sure what to think about this blood type information because she had been down the diet path so many times before. But Gennie made her mind up to go for it and enrolled in the program.

When she started, her body fat was approximately 42 percent, and she was on medication for high cholesterol—which tested at 250 (with the medication)! After eating correctly for her blood type for one month, Gennie's cholesterol dropped to 200. By the end of her second month she had lost twenty-three pounds and gone down three dress sizes. In addition, her cholesterol was down to 180. After three and a half months, Gennie had dropped a total of thirty pounds and gone down eight dress sizes. Her cholesterol is now steady at 160, a level she never was able to get close to with all the other dieting plans.

Gennie went to her doctor throughout those three months to be monitored. Her doctor was completely amazed at her progress and improved health. She told Gennie to keep up whatever it was that she was doing.

Of course, the results of eating for blood type will vary from individual to individual. But when we use the right tools, we can experience fantastic results. Helping people become healthy and stay that way is a God-given passion of mine. I'm not going to force good health and happiness on you, but if you want it, it's there for you. Every time students like Gennie come back with a good bill of health from their doctors, it makes my day. I am very pleased and happy for them.

Ever since I discovered this lifestyle of eating, I have been promoting it (along with exercising) in a big way. I now have statistics on hundreds of people who have come through the doors of our studio. All this information shows that an exercise program combined with blood type dietary changes can benefit anyone.

Most who follow the blood type approach to eating say they

feel free to eat, generally are not hungry and have lost their cravings for sweets. Most say this lifestyle of eating for their blood type is realistic enough to be able to follow all the time. And the best reward is that they feel good!

Abandoning the old myths and embracing the new truths is the key to being set free.

3

A Clean Invironment

*For you created my inmost being;
you knit me together in my mother's womb.
I praise you because I am fearfully and
wonderfully made; your works are
wonderful, I know that full well.*
—PSALM 139:13–14

PILLAR THREE

7

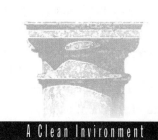

ELIMINATION—THE
UNMENTIONABLE SUBJECT

Pollution! You've read about it in all the newspapers and magazines. You've watched it on the six o'clock news. You've breathed it on the freeways. Pollution is a serious ecological problem of global magnitude that affects every human being.

Unless we clean up our environment and stop polluting it, we will bring ill-health and even imminent death to ourselves and our children. The forests, trees, plants and wildlife, as well as the ozone layer, are all slowly dying. Our planet has become a sick environment for man, and soon we will no longer be able to live the healthy life we knew many years ago.

While we all should do our part for improving our environment and surroundings, this Pillar is not about our environment. It is about our "invironment." The term *invironment* was coined by Dr. Albert Zehr. Dr. Zehr states, "While the environment is the atmosphere and surroundings in which we live, the 'invironment' is the atmosphere and surroundings inside of us."[1] Just as our environment is being plagued by pollution, so is our invironment also.

Unless we do two things—stop polluting and clean up the existing pollution—we will be faced with unnecessary health-related illnesses and eventually have a less than acceptable quality of life—to the point that we experience premature death.

Sound rather serious, doesn't it? Well, it certainly is! Once you learn the crucial role your invironment plays regarding enhancing your health or destroying it, you will be motivated to stop polluting it and instead clean it up.

If you were to ask my mother what stood out about me as a child, she would tell you that it was my curiosity. I always wanted to know what was going on inside my toys, what made them work. My goal for this Pillar of Health is to raise your curiosity to a level that you will understand the importance of keeping your invironment as unpolluted as possible.

So let's take a trip through the digestive system and see how it works.

THE PATH OF A MOUTHFUL OF FOOD

ELIMINATION IS ONE of the most important yet probably the least understood bodily functions. That's probably because it's not something we talk about every day. In fact, it's a taboo subject—one we avoid. Who wants to talk about waste, bowels and parasites? We'd rather talk about beautiful, healthy and pleasant things. But as we'll discover, the elimination process, when functioning properly, leads to beauty and health. And when functioning improperly, it can lead to lack of energy at best, and sickness and disease at worst. So it's worth putting aside the taboos and talking about it, don't you think?

When you swallow a mouthful of food, it goes to your stomach to be converted to a semiliquid form called *chyme*. After the food (chyme) leaves your stomach, it travels through the small intestine. The chyme passes from the small intestine into the colon through the ileocecal valve. The colon, a large muscular organ five feet long, is located at the end of your digestive tract.

70

HEALTH **FACT** BOX

> The colon has three basic functions:
> 1. To absorb water and electrolytes from the chyme
> 2. To move waste material out of the body
> 3. To store the waste until it is evacuated

Imagine your colon being like a curvy roller-coaster. The passengers (chyme—consisting of food, water, liver excretions and so forth) enter the roller-coaster car, which starts at the bottom (the cecum). The colon begins to move the car up the ascending colon with involuntary wavelike contractions, a process called peristalsis. Billions of friendly bacteria in our colon break down some of the materials we can't digest, and from this process come nutrients like vitamin K and a few of the B vitamins. This bacterial team also breaks down some of the protein into less complex substances.

When the car reaches the hepatic flexure at the top of the ascending colon, it does a 90-degree turn and goes across the transverse colon, still climbing to a higher level. From there the car does another 90-degree turn at the splenic flexure and heads straight down the descending colon to the end of the ride at the sigmoid colon and the rectum.[2]

During the digestive process the chyme is moved through the colon by the peristaltic muscular action in the colon walls. In this process some positive bacteria and moisture are withdrawn. The

71

HEALTH **FACT** BOX

In the past several years many health authorities have agreed that most illnesses are linked directly to either a blockage in the colon or poor bowel function. Well-known bowel specialist V. E. Irons claims, "In my opinion there is only one real disease, and that disease is autointoxication—the body poisoning itself. It's the filth in our system that kills us. So, I'm convinced that unless you clean out your colon you will never regain vibrant health."[3]

Dr. Norman Walker also states, "Good health not only regenerates and builds the cells and tissues which constitute your physical body, but also is involved in the processes by which the waste matter, the undigested food, is eliminated from your body to prevent corruption in the form of fermentation and putrefaction. This corruption, if retained and allowed to accumulate in the body, prevents any possibility of attaining any degree of vibrant health."[4]

Dr. Walker concludes by saying, "Not to cleanse the colon is like having the entire garbage collection staff in your city go on strike for days on end. The accumulation of garbage in the streets creates putrid, odoriferous, unhealthy gases which are dispersed into the atmosphere."[5]

matter that begins its downward journey through the descending colon is called feces. Toxicity and waste from your blood as well as putrefying bacteria are carried in the fecal matter to the sigmoid colon, the rectum and then out of the body.

72

Elimination–the Unmentionable Subject

If the colon is healthy and operating normally, it will eliminate the toxic waste materials easily and regularly without strain. But if your colon is not in good operating condition, it will not eliminate properly. This causes those toxins in the feces to build up in your system and begin damaging and destroying your health.

THE COLON AND YOUR HEALTH

THINK FOR A moment back to elementary school. Do you remember mixing flour and water to make paste? That paste enabled you to glue paper ornaments together or glue cut-outs to a page.

A similar paste-like substance can build up in your colon. If the food selections you make are not compatible to your blood type, if they are not in their freshest state and full of roughage but instead are processed, or if they are dairy, they are difficult for your colon to move through the digestive tract. Consequently, a slime builds up on the porous walls of the colon, which actually plasters the walls like paste.

As the buildup continues over the years, your body can no longer absorb the nutrients and nutritional supplements through those walls. Often, because of the buildup on the inner walls, there is barely enough space for food and fecal material to pass through. Believe it or not, most people are walking around malnourished— even those who eat regularly and take their vitamins. They lack energy because their colons are clogged. According to Dr. Norman Walker, a specialist in colon health, "The consequent result is a starvation of which we are not conscious, but which causes old age and senility to race toward us with the throttle wide open."[6]

"In the fifty years I've spent helping people to overcome disability and disease, it has become crystal clear that poor bowel management lies at the root of most people's health problems. In treating over 300,000 patients, it is the bowel that invariably has to be cared for first before effective healing can take place," says Dr. Bernard Jensen.[7]

Frighteningly, your internal digestive, absorption and elimination

HEALTH **FACT** BOX

Several unnecessary illnesses are common today because of the conditions of our colons. Hopefully, recognizing them will raise your level of awareness and motivate you to clean your invironment and avoid the dismal consequences.[8]

- Constipation—caused primarily by insufficient dietary fiber
- Diverticulosis—a pouch-like sack or ballooning in the intestines, caused by increased internal pressure and weakening of the bowel wall
- Diverticulitis—inflamed diverticula
- Colitis—inflammation of the colon, also known as irritable bowel or spastic colon, when the inner lining of the colon becomes inflamed
- Hemorrhoids—dilated veins in the anus and rectum
- Stricture—Chronic narrowing of the colon passage due to inflammation
- Prolapsed colon—falling of the transverse colon because of accumulated waste material and general deterioration of colon health as a result of poor colon hygiene

system can be turned into a garbage dump that will pollute your body and weaken and destroy your health.

When the chyme and fecal matter cannot move regularly through the colon and be disposed of, they ferment and putrefy

HEALTH **FACT** BOX

There are several important steps that you can take to keep your colon healthy. These include:

- Get enough fiber daily.
- Drink pure water only.
- Maintain a healthy low-fat, high-fiber diet.
- Get regular moderate exercise.
- Reduce as much stress as possible in your life.
- Supplement your diet with friendly bacteria, such as in nonfat, plain or vanilla yogurt.
- Periodically cleanse your colon.

just as if a sewage system were backed up. Think of the environmental health problems that would exist if the sewer system in your city was backed up and ignored by the sanitation department. It wouldn't take too many days before the sewer system became a cesspool, polluting the entire environment and causing parasitic infestation and disease. Your city would become extremely toxic—not an acceptable environment in which to live.

Well, the very same results occur when your digestive system is not kept operating properly. Many people are in a constant state of fatigue, lethargy and sickness because of their neglected interior sanitation system.

AUTOINTOXICATION

DO YOU EXPERIENCE the blahs—not just once in a while, but day after

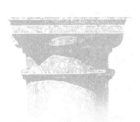

Many people are in a constant state of fatigue, lethargy and sickness because of their neglected interior sanitation system.

day? You might exercise regularly, eat healthy foods and even take dietary supplements to ensure proper nutrient intake. But still you feel less healthy than you should for all the good preventative steps you are taking. Well, you could possibly be suffering from autointoxication.

If your colon is congested and has been plastered for a long time, it probably is not functioning normally. In fact, it cannot function normally! Your body cannot rid itself of the rotting fecal matter because it's impacted onto the walls, and that slows down your body's ability to eliminate efficiently. Ultimately your congested colon is actually poisoning you and producing toxicity throughout your entire body.

This condition of your colon also affects your body's ability to absorb nutrients properly. In fact, the small amount it is absorbing is toxic because a congested colon is polluted and very toxic. Your entire digestive system becomes a toxic dump, and these toxins are carried via the blood stream to other areas of your body, introducing you to an another entire host of health problems.

According to Dr. Bernard Jensen, autointoxication is "the result of faulty bowel functioning which produces undesirable consequences in the body and is the root cause of many of today's illnesses and diseases."9

The colon seems to be able to endure this infectious and toxic condition without much pain because it lacks nerve endings. Unfortunately, many of these abnormalities are allowed to develop because they go unnoticed.

While growing up, I would hear my relatives or people in general talk about their spastic colon or other colon problems. Many

Elimination—the Unmentionable Subject

people have colon problems like that, plus more. Harvey W. Kellog, M.D., says, "Of the 22,000 operations I personally performed, I never found a single normal colon, and of the 100,000 performed under my jurisdiction not over 6 percent were normal."[10]

According to Dr. Walker, "If a person has eaten processed, fried and overcooked foods, devitalized starches, sugar and excessive amounts of salts, his colon cannot possibly be efficient, even if he should have a bowel movement two to three times a day."[11]

This Pillar is very important for everyone to maintain, but it is usually overlooked because of the undesirability of the topic. Hopefully, you can get past that mind-set and realize the importance of keeping the colon operating in tip-top condition.

8

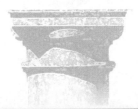

INVASION
OF THE PARASITES

Approximately three hundred types of parasites thrive in the intestinal tracts of people in America today.[1] It is quite possible that you are walking around town, a human buffet for tiny little invaders that did not receive your VIP invitation.

June Wiles, Ph.D., and parasite expert, stated, "Parasites are vermin that steal your food, drink your blood and leave their excrement in your body to be reabsorbed into the blood stream as nourishment."[2]

Whether a microscopic single-cell parasite or a four-inch worm, these little parasites love to eat whatever the host is eating—but they are first in line. After they are thoroughly fed, we get what is left over, mainly in the form of excrement.

Parasites can also become your unwelcome guests through shaking hands and playing with your pets. They can be transferred by adults, children and food handlers. You can get parasites by eating uncooked meats or raw fruits and veggies.

When I was in Cancún, Mexico, with Planet Hollywood, I ate a Caesar salad. The next day we flew to London, and I had stomach and intestinal problems for almost two weeks because of a parasite I picked up from the salad.

HEALTH**FACT**BOX

Parasites come in all types—pinworms, tape-worms, hookworms, roundworms, ringworms and *Giardia lamblia,* a tiny microscopic parasite being studied by scientists today in America. "One out of every four in the world is infected by roundworms, which cause fever, cough, and intestinal problems. One quarter of the world's people have hookworms, which can cause anemia and abdominal pain. A third of a billion people suffer from the abdominal pain and diarrhea caused by whipworms."[3]

Parasites are easily passed around by millions of people each day just by coming in contact with one another. And if you consider the millions of people who eat at restaurants every day, you can see how parasitic contact can become overwhelming. Usually if one member of your family has them, then everyone will get them.

Among children in temperate climates the pinworm is the most common parasite. Overcrowded schools and day-care centers aid in passing these parasites around. These conditions have caused an increase in pinworm infestation in children. One child in six having pinworms used to be the norm, but now this infestation is up to an astounding 90 percent of children in America.[4]

While there are more than three hundred varieties of parasites, only about twenty-five varieties can be seen without a microscope. Those that can be seen without a microscope include pinworms, hookworms, roundworms and tapeworms. These critters build colonies in the rectum and colon and cause them to be irritated and raw.[5]

In the Southern states, the hookworm is most common. This uninvited body destroyer causes abdominal pain, diarrhea, malnutrition, apathy, anemia and even underdevelopment in children.

The problem of parasites is much more widespread than the health professionals ever dreamed it could be. Centers for Disease Control experts point out that doctors are at a loss when it comes to the diseases brought on by parasites because their training and schooling is very limited on parasitic infestations.[6] Doctors are reluctant to admit to the microbial epidemics like parasites and clogged colons. Most people are ignorant of the health problems that can be caused by parasites.

It is a medically known fact that impacted, clogged intestines and junk-filled and sugar-filled colons are the two major causes for the epidemic breakout of parasites. This condition of your invironment makes a perfect place for all worms of all sizes to thrive.

Intestinal parasites and worms can cause you to be sick. For instance, if you are housing *Giardia lamblia,* you may end up doubled over with abdominal pain or vomiting, belching, feverish and exploding diarrhea. Unfortunately, antibiotics do not affect the *Giardia.*

Having intestinal parasites or worms may also cause you to have a greater susceptibility to weight problems because the parasitic infestation is due to the accumulation of undigested food and impacted food. That condition lends itself to the parasites building colonies, which break down and destroy the normal digestive functions. Consequently the body cannot assimilate or digest foods properly.

Many parasites do not penetrate the intestinal wall, but they leave your blood stream full of their excrement. If they cannot enter your intestinal region, they can still dump toxins in your body and can challenge your immune system.

Invasion of the Parasites

TRANSIT TIME

TRANSIT TIME IS the amount of time it should take for a healthy colon to transport the nutrients into the body for nourishment and then dispose of the toxic waste that remains. The volume of food and liquids ingested as well as the condition of the colon determines transit time. In a healthy colon the transit time should be no more than sixteen to twenty-four hours. Elimination should occur once after each full meal. If the body takes longer than the normal transit time to eliminate the waste, then toxic buildup begins.

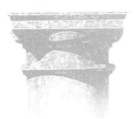

It is a medically known fact that impacted, clogged intestines and junk-filled and sugar-filled colons are the two major causes for the epidemic breakout of parasites.

Once toxic buildup occurs, your digestive tract becomes a real breeding ground for parasites. These little guys are looking for a home to raise their families—and they love to multiply and produce lots of kids.

The faster the roller-coaster ride, the less time these parasites have to multiply. The average incubation period for a parasite is thirty-six hours, so if your roller-coaster car is traveling at the prescribed sixteen to twenty-four hours, then you are in good shape. On the other hand, if your colon's transit time is that of the average American's, then you have serious problems. That's because the average transit time for people in America is ninety-six hours![7]

Dr. Tom Spies, recipient of the American Medical Association's (AMA) Distinguished Service Award, reminds us, "All the chemicals used in the body—except for the oxygen we breathe and the water we drink—are taken through food."[8] The choices of food selections we make have a direct link to the way the bowel responds. Studies have shown that the regular intake of refined carbohydrates or sugars and the lack of most Americans to include sufficient fiber in

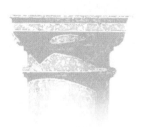

The only way to cleanse the colon is with natural ingredients.

their diet slows down the transit time, increases the buildup of waste and fecal matter and promotes putrefactive bacteria.

Remember, your colon is your sewage system, and you cannot afford to neglect it. Through neglect or ignorance thousands of people suffer from diverticulitis, irritable bowel syndrome, cancer of the colon and many other chronic diseases because of the poor sanitation service they are giving their bodies. An unhealthy colon impacted with sugars, burgers, fries and white-flour products is at the root of these poor health problems.

At the turn of the twentieth century a health survey was taken involving approximately 110 different nations. Our country ranked thirteenth from the top for good health. Recently, a similar survey was taken of seventy-nine countries, and the United States ranked seventy-ninth.[9] We're a sick people, and we are not giving our children a good shot at their future when we just sit back and do nothing about it.

Many medical experts consider it myth that a plaque-coated colon or parasitic infestation could be directly linked to illness, disease and sickness. This attitude may be due to the fact that there is no patented medicine or drug for quick relief of an impacted colon. In fact, medicines can't unclog an impacted intestinal tract or colon.

You might want to consider that your colon and intestinal tract may be totally coated with plaque. That along with parasites may be making you feel lousy, weak and unhealthy. Do you have foul breath, feel achy, have sore joints or regular headaches? Then there is a good chance that your colon needs some invironmental cleansing.

Perhaps by this point you are screaming, "What can I do?" The only way to cleanse the colon is with natural ingredients.

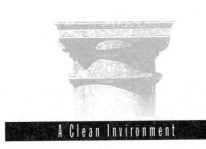

9

A Clean Invironment

CLEANSING THE COLON

Several years ago my wife and I decided to make colon cleansing a part of our overall health and fitness program. We understood the value and importance of the colon and how it functioned. We learned the important role it plays in keeping our bodies free of both slime and parasites, so we decided to do winter and spring cleansings of our invironments.

SPRING CLEANING

THE COLON CLEANSE program that we believe is the most thorough and effective is a two-week, three-phase program. (See Appendix A for information on this program.) Although several cleansing programs as well as self-designed programs are available, I want to tell you about the one we use as an example of what they are like. My hope is that you will discover they are not frightening and that you will decide to try one.

The first phase of our two-week colon cleanse is a seven-day period in which we take a pouch of multi-nutrients and herbs both in the morning and in the evening. We don't make any eating adjustments during those first seven days. The nutrients start breaking down all the mucus that has been building up in the colon wall. Parasites are also killed, and their dwelling places are eliminated.

During the first phase I notice some rumblings in my colon, but that is just the cleansing taking place. This particular program does not work like an herbal laxative, so we do not have to worry about hanging around the restrooms for two weeks.

The second phase lasts for four days and requires a juice fast. All solids are avoided during this phase. We mix packets of powder with juice four times a day. This phase really makes things start happening!

During this phase the powder mixed with the juice has a powerful action that actually scrubs the porous walls of the colon to open up its ability to absorb again. The clay in this powder also works like a sponge and absorbs the mucoids and parasites that have been destroyed. It can also absorb up to forty times its weight in toxic matter. This prevents the toxins from being reabsorbed into the body as they are traveling out of the colon. The scrubbed and cleaned out colon will then allow elimination of built-up fecal matter much easier.

During this phase we sometimes experience abrupt reactions to the cleansing process. The first time Lori went through this phase, she broke out with canker sores in her mouth. They lasted only a couple of days, but it was the way her body released the toxins that were built up in her system. I experienced about three days of headaches, which disappeared quickly. Others have felt weak and unmotivated for a day or two when the body is attempting to release the toxic buildup and free up its system. But after going through colon cleansing two or three times, the body reacts less and less abruptly, because it is cleaner and has less toxicity to remove.

During this second phase, we try to minimize our exercise, work and physical activities. We just relax the best we can. If it is impossible to get away from work or from our normal hectic schedule, we still can go through the colon cleansing rather easily.

Lori and I find that this four-day juice fast is a great time for meditating and praying. We often choose an area in our lives upon which we want to focus during that fast period. That gives us a quality time of coming back into harmony and balance. A time of isolation from the rest of the world just to get still will do wonders for the soul as well as the body.

Many people have difficulty fasting because they normally eat to satisfy an emotion, not for nourishment. I have been told by some of my clients that they could not imagine going a day without eating. I believe this is more psychological reasoning than fear of starvation. This particular fast is a juice fast, so we are not completely going without nourishment. Plus, the juices are satisfying.

The third phase of the colon cleanse is simply returning to normal eating while still taking morning and evening packets of nutrients for restoration and strengthening of the colon. But because we are virtually empty and yet carrying that powder clay from the juice fast stage, our bodies are ready to eliminate what has been stored there for months and even years.

After the cleanse we feel brand spanking new! For the first day or two, we eat foods that are easy to break down, staying away from meats or proteins and instead eating complex carbohydrates. The colon has just had its spring or winter cleaning and is sensitive to food and pollution.

If you try a colon cleanse, you will feel like a new person, too. When the colon has been scrubbed clean and the parasites and mucoids have been removed, the body will absorb foods much more efficiently. After a colon cleansing, your energy will increase, your mental alertness will be keener, and you will have satisfaction of mind that you have done the right thing for your health.

My brother Bob, who had been dealing with headaches every day for years, found complete and total relief from his headaches

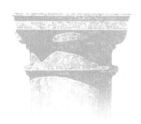

After a colon cleansing, your energy will increase, your mental alertness will be keener, and you will have satisfaction of mind that you have done the right thing for your health.

after one cleansing. Some people who have used this program have reported eliminating seeds that they hadn't eaten for over six months, as well as worms up to four inches long.

Keep in mind that if you do not have a bowel movement three times daily, then you are considered clinically constipated. If you eat two or three meals a day and only eliminate once every two or three days, where do you think all that waste is? It's impacted in your colon. Think about babies—all they do is eat and poop, eat and poop, just like clockwork. That's because their colon is clean and running the way it should.

I have described the colon cleanse that works best for us. But if you go to your local health food store, you will find many products available to cleanse the colon. Some people take coffee enemas, and other have colonics done by professionals. Choose whichever method fits you best, but choose to cleanse your colon.

CLEANSING THROUGH ELIMINATING THE FOUR WHITES

IN MY EXPERIENCE as a fitness professional and nutrition guide I have noticed again and again that most people choose the wrong foods as their staples. Generally speaking, the majority of their selections come from what I call the "four whites"—white flour, refined sugar, salt and fat. Allowing these foods to remain in your diet over time will cause destruction to your superstructure similar to the destruction that termites do to a house.

Cleansing the Colon

Eliminate white flour

People cannot easily digest the white flour that breads, bagels, rolls, pastas and even pretzels are made of. Though these foods are common, they are not good for your body. White flour in any product is dead flour, and it provides empty, useless calories. Let me show you what I mean.

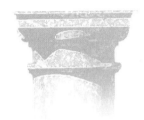

In obvious acknowledgment that good things have been removed, manufacturers then add some synthetic nutrients and call it "fortified, enriched" flour.

God created the wheat in the fields perfect in its total composition. It lacked nothing and did not need to be fortified. The problem flour—white flour—is flour that fell into the hands of the food manufacturers. In the process of getting that beautiful white flour to your dinner table, all fiber is stripped from it. During its destructive journey a bleaching process is necessary, which destroys the nutrients. In obvious acknowledgment that good things have been removed, manufacturers then add some synthetic nutrients and call it "fortified, enriched" flour.

Many innocent shoppers assume that everything on the grocery shelves is good for them. But that's not true.

White flour is a major contributor to weight problems, low blood sugar and the inability to fight the good fight against the sugar monster. The body treats white flour as sugar; when it is eaten too often and too much, the body experiences an over-insulin response, which contributes to slowing down its metabolism (the very thing you need running at high speed for weight management). Consequently, white flour causes us to get fat.

Besides getting fat, our bodies are not getting the nutrients or fiber that were originally in the wheat when it was in the Garden.

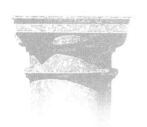

Refined sugar is not digestible; it contributes to tooth decay, obesity, depression, hyperactivity, hypoglycemia, weakness, cancers and much more.

Over time, often at a slow pace, the body breaks down because it hasn't been receiving the nutrients it requires. Last but certainly not least, this "wonder food" has clogged the colon and allowed it to become the hostess of the most-est parasites in town.

Perhaps you thought junk foods were limited to candies, cakes and chocolates. Well, white flour and white-flour products must be included in this category. Do yourself and your family a favor and do not buy any more white flour products. Try eating Ezekiel bread (sprouted grains and wheat) instead, which is compatible with everybody's blood type. You can get it at your local health food store in the freezer section. Also, try buckwheat, barley flour, spelt, millet or 100 percent rye bread.

If you eat wheat bread, keep it to a minimum. But if you are a blood type O or B, eliminate it completely. If you love pasta, try spelt, rice flour and Jerusalem artichoke pasta as alternatives.

Eliminate refined sugar

Refined sugar is basic table sugar, which is found in candies, pastries, cookies, pies, sodas, sweetened iced tea, doughnuts, ice cream—and the list goes on and on. I'm sure you're familiar with all these good-tasting ingestibles. (Did you notice I didn't call them foods?) Many processed foods contain a high amount of sugar, too.

Refined sugar is not digestible; it contributes to tooth decay, obesity, depression, hyperactivity, hypoglycemia, weakness, cancers and much more. Does this sound like something you would recommend to someone you love—even yourself?

Interesting, isn't it, that parents will reward their children with sweet goodies for performing well or obeying. This only sets their children's health into a downward spin. Too many sweets can cause kids to become hyper and out of control. Then in desperation, parents accept prescriptions for antidepressants and hyperactivity medications for their children.

Here's a tip if you are a soda drinker: Get off of it. Come off immediately or come off slowly, but do come off soda. Replace every can of soda you eliminate with a glass of water. If you need that fizzy feeling in your throat, then have some sparkling water. It even comes in various flavors in case plain sparking water is too boring for you.

HEALTH FACT BOX

Many of the clients I have counseled seemed to be hooked on soda. I had a client who used to drink ten to twenty 12-ounce cans of soda a day. By the way, that is about 450 cans per month. With 12 tablespoons of table sugar in each can, that equates to 180 tablespoons of sugar per day, or 5,400 tablespoons a month.[1] That is just like adding a slew of chemicals and some water to a 10-pound bag of sugar and drinking it every month. Do you think she had headaches or a difficult time losing weight? You better believe it—that and more!

Moderate salt intake

Salt is also called sodium chloride because about 40 percent of salt is sodium and the rest is chloride. If you eat a diet high in salt, it is also usually high in sodium. Sodium is a double-edged sword. It is a key element for maintaining proper bodily functions, and when

89

taken in normal amounts, it regulates proper metabolic function. But when the levels of sodium are elevated, the body begins retaining water to create an equilibrium between sodium and water. Likewise when the body water is low (say, after exercise), the brains signals the thirst sensation so the person will drink water and bring back the equilibrium between sodium and water.

The average American diet contains too much salt. When the levels of sodium are high, the water level is also high. Excess fluid in the body must be removed by the kidneys. Over time, this overload on the kidneys may cause health problems such as kidney damage or even failure. Along with kidney problems, the retention of water may stress the heart by increasing the volume of blood it needs to pump. High blood pressure may be directly associated with high sodium consumption as well.

As an alternative for that salty taste bud of yours, consider using sea salt or kelp.

HEALTH FACT BOX

According to most research, as well as the Food and Drug Administration (FDA), the Recommended Daily Allowance (RDA) for sodium intake is 1,100 to 3,300 milligrams per day. One teaspoon of salt contains about 2,000 milligrams. Yet the average American diet consists of 4,000 to 8,000 milligrams per day.[2]

Eliminate the bad fats

Not all fat is the same. Some fats are harmful when over-consumed, yet others enhance your health. To understand this, let's look at the three types of fat: saturated fat, monounsaturated fat and polyunsaturated fat.

Saturated fats are typically solid at room temperature. Most of these fats come from animal sources, such as red meats and whole dairy products like butter and cheese. Vegetable oils high in saturated fats are coconut oil, palm oil, palm kernel oil, cocoa butter and hydrogenated vegetable oils.

Saturated fats tend to raise your total cholesterol count. They are difficult to digest and play a major role in the development of coronary heart disease.

Monounsaturated fats are generally vegetable and remain liquid at room temperature. A primary source of mono-unsaturated fats is olive oil. These were formerly termed "neutral fats," meaning they were neither good nor bad for people. But recent studies have shown an association with lowering the bad cholesterol (LDL) without lowering the good cholesterol (HDL).

Polyunsaturated fats are usually vegetable and stay liquid at room temperature also. These are the preferred fats to ingest. They are easily digested and act to lower LDL (bad cholesterol) values. Safflower oil, cottonseed oil, soybean oil and corn oil are some examples of polyunsaturated fats. Generally, Americans are advised to take no more than 10 percent of their daily calories in polyunsaturated fats.[3]

Remember, when making any dietary changes, make them gradually. Try one or two changes at a time, then add others. This will ensure long-term success.

CLEANSING THROUGH
EATING FOR YOUR BLOOD TYPE

EATING THE RIGHT foods can help eliminate conditions in the digestive system that are derogatory to our health. By eating foods that are compatible to our blood types (and avoiding those that aren't), we can actually find relief from digestive disorders, discomfort and illnesses.

Certain foods are treated by a particular blood type as a poison. They interfere with the normal digestive process. But those same foods will be treated as a medicine by another blood type.

Eating foods that are compatible to your blood type will allow your body to go through a detoxification period because of the blood type association with the wall of the digestive track. You will experience a tremendous relief in the digestive tract, and you will be able to assimilate your food more efficiently. Consequently, you will have little to no gastrointestinal problems. You will have a greater sense of being satisfied after eating because of the improved digestion and absorption abilities. There will also be fewer opportunities for parasitic infestation to take hold.

And all that comes just by making food selections that are compatible to your blood type.

Colon Health Is Critical

IN THEIR BOOK *Cleansing the Body and the Colon for a Happier and Healthier You,* Teresa Schumacher and Toni Lund tell the following story: One day the body organs got together and decided to have a board meeting. Here's what went on behind closed doors. There was intense discussion to determine who was the most important part of the body.

The brain was the first to speak. "Without me, nothing would be accomplished."

Then the heart spoke up. "Without me pumping blood to your brain, you could not function."

The arms laughed. "You're both wrong. Without me to put food in the mouth, nothing would work."

Cleansing the Colon

The stomach said, "Without me, your food would not digest."

The lungs bellowed back, "Without us, you could not breathe."

The eyes blinked, "Without me, you could not see."

The kidneys snorted, "Without me, you could not detoxify and eliminate."

Then the colon meekly spoke up. "I am important. You need me to eliminate all of the garbage from your systems."

Everyone laughed and made fun of him. "How can you be as important as we are? You're just a smelly old sewer." The poor colon—his feelings were hurt. He turned away and thought, *I'll show them.* He shut down! Then he sat back and watched what happened.

The brain was stupefied.

The heart's beat was weak and irregular.

The arms were weak and couldn't move.

The lungs gave in to shallow breathing.

The eyes became clouded.

The kidneys quit.

The colon looked around and decided it was time to call another meeting. It wasn't too lively this time, but everyone was in total agreement—the colon was the most important organ![4]

The information regarding this mighty Pillar of Health might seem somewhat gross at first, but ignoring the condition of your invironment will not change the sobering importance of your colon. The body that you were given to live in is a very precise piece of machinery that requires constant attention. Your body is in and of itself so incredibly intertwined that it is impossible to ever assume that each gland, system and organ will somehow take care of itself. When one breaks down, the others are affected.

We Americans have all the advantages of technological advancements, new medical discoveries, procedures and remedies, plus advancements in dietary and nutritional research. We should be the healthiest people on Planet Earth. On the contrary—we are a very unhealthy people. The solution to the problem lies with each of us not being willing to settle for a standard of living that includes laziness, empathy or mediocrity.

My purpose is not to suggest that your marvelously designed body is in need of some external concoction or methodology to improve its own natural and innate ability to survive a lifetime. But the damage that you cause to your body by turning the other way or thinking that some day it will improve on its own is formidable. That kind of thinking is responsible for keeping your physical body in an unhealthy condition and robbing you of a life that can be enjoyed to its fullest.

Your life is the superstructure that requires the highest level of optimum bodily function and performance. This Pillar of Health is unequivocally the one that supports your entire superstructure. If the colon is neglected, overlooked or abused, there is absolutely no hope for any life that resembles what you were created to enjoy.

So start today to keep your colon in tip-top shape!

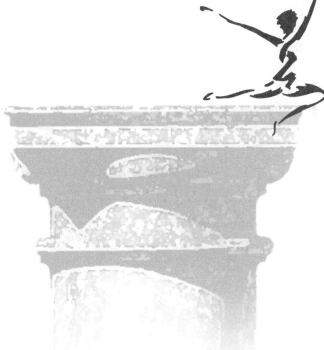

A Strong Immune System

*My people are destroyed
from lack of knowledge.*
—Hosea 4:6

4

PILLAR FOUR

10

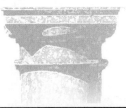

THE IMMUNE SYSTEM: ARMED FORCES AGAINST INVADERS

When I was a child, my brother Bob and I played the board game Risk with our friends. From the onset of the game, players are surrounded by invading armies out to overtake them. We used our armies to attack the territories of others and to protect our territories from attack. The key to protecting our own territory from invaders was building up our armies so they outnumbered the enemy.

So it is in the real world. Ever since you took your first breath, your body has been attacked by various invaders trying to get inside your body. These invaders are turned away by your army, the immune system. Without that army, your body would be extremely vulnerable to sickness and disease.

Every human body is equipped with an amazing capacity to protect and preserve itself. All of us who are in pursuit of a life of vitality and good health must tend to this Pillar of Health. It is our own health protector and is necessary to support a strong, healthy and disease-free superstructure.

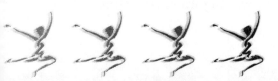

Seven Pillars of Health

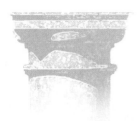

Ever since you took your first breath, your body has been attacked by various invaders trying to get inside your body.

Under Attack!

Encased within your body's largest organ, your skin, is a massive collection of sixty trillion cells. These cells are different from each other and are uniquely arranged to form the varying organs and systems, which, when all working together in harmony, allow your body to function properly. So keeping happy, healthy cells is imperative for healthy living.

But in order for us to survive, let alone live healthier lives, our cells must be nourished, cared for and maintained to function properly in their biochemical realm. The cells must also be protected from the continual attacks of their enemies. Picture your body as the universal ballroom where those sixty trillion cells get together and dance perfectly, and you will see why they are so adamant about not allowing any uninvited guests to their functions.

The problem is, your body, like the players in Risk, is living in an extremely hostile and unforgiving environment. From your first day on this planet, your body has been surrounded by vicious enemies that are continually trying to find ways to enter your body, to harass and disturb your party. You must be able to recognize these enemies in order to resist their attempt to crash your body's "Health Party" and avoid the diseases they bring with them. These enemies include yeast and fungi, which attempt to establish colonies, reproduce and eventually cause your body to decompose. Also on the uninvited guest list are viruses that afflict your body with illness and disease. And of course, this list would not be complete without bacteria, which putrefy and spread death. As you can see, we are walking around in enemy territory.

The Immune System: Armed Forces Against Invaders

If you think these enemy attacks are the only means by which health can be ruined, you are wrong. Cancer, for instance, occurs when our cells reproduce themselves uncontrollably. The polluted air we breathe, the polluted water we drink and the processed foods we eat that contain preservatives and additives also damage our cells and weaken our immune system. We cannot escape this endless warfare of invaders battling against our immune systems.

Many times my profession calls for me to travel. Just by boarding an airplane I can come into contact with global germs. And that's not taking into consideration the physical contact I may have with people from around the world, which can expose me to a large number of viruses, fungi and bacteria. Have you attended a formal event, church service or a public event where someone shook your hand right after sneezing in their own? It might have been healthier to salute that person instead!

The very fact that you and I are alive is proof that our immune systems are actively working on our behalf. But this Immune System Pillar must be shored up and fortified. With such a variety of enemy forces marching against our borders, it is absolutely necessary to build up a strong defensive army to protect our own cells and then to identify, seek out and destroy all intruders.

Have you ever wondered why some of your family members seem to catch everything that comes along, while others do not? Why does your grandmother—who suffers with heart problems—and the old man up the street—with emphysema—and the toddlers in the day-care class you teach seem to be the first ones to catch the flu and other viruses going around? Why does the body try to reject the transplanted organ that could give it new life? Or why do kids get chicken pox and other childhood diseases only once? The answers can be found by studying our immune system.

How the Immune Army Operates

"Seek and destroy" is a military offensive strategy usually used by the infantry. And that is exactly what your immune system does in response to an attack. At the first sign of an invader, such as bacteria, the immune system sounds the alarm, which alerts the defense system to seek and destroy the enemy.

Patrol vehicles

The immune system has a tremendously sophisticated method of determining whether a substance is foreign or friendly. Not only is it able to recognize millions of enemy molecules attempting an attack, but it can produce molecules and cells to form a line of

HEALTH FACT BOX

The immune system is as complex in its structure as the brain and nervous system. It can distinguish the enemy from its own "invited guests." It can remember previous experiences—like a round of chicken pox—and prevent that experience from happening again. And it has at its command a sophisticated array of weapons.

impenetrable defense to counterattack the enemy and drive it off. Chemical markers, or antigens, are found on every cell in the body. Blood type antigens are some of the most powerful antigens in the body. The blood type antigen identifies whether the invader is a friend or foe by checking out the antigen located on the invader.

Lymphocytes are a type of white blood cells that actually patrol the circulatory system and the areas of fluid immediately surrounding the cells. They are the main functional cells of the immune system.[1] They consist mostly of T cells, responsible for cell immunity, and B cells, responsible for antibody production.

T cells travel widely throughout the body. They help the body to defend against foreign substances, and they surround damaged or diseased body cells.

The B cells, too, are called into battle. Specialized B cells produce antibodies, and these antibodies function like anti-aircraft missiles, firing their antibodies on invading enemy viruses and diseases. These B cell antibodies join forces with the T cells to surround the diseased cells and to destroy them.

While this internal war is raging on your behalf, you might experience some soreness or even pain in your joints as well as inflammation and redness in the lymph nodes. When these symptoms occur, don't panic; it is just your body's way of reacting to biochemical casualties taking place. It's actually a wonderful indication that your system is doing its job.

The clean-up crew

Another group of white blood cells named "macrophages" are then recruited into action. Macrophages are large immune cells that devour invading pathogens and other intruders. The modus operandi of these guys is to eat everything in sight that is covered with antibodies. Then, after they eat, they explode. The circulatory system then cleans up the mess by carrying the deceased to the elimination department.

The amazing immune system always keeps an adequate supply of antibodies in reserve ready for the next attack. Some of the lymphocytes have a good memory; in case there is ever another encounter with that flu virus or other disease, the alarm will sound immediately, and victory will be sweet one more time. This is what we refer to as immunity to a disease. It is why children seldom catch the same childhood disease twice.

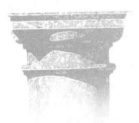

The strength of the immune response to the invader is dependent upon the strength and condition of the host's immune system.

Military police

It's no secret how vicious the immune system can become, but at the same time it can be very sensitive. In fact, it will turn on itself and attack the body's own cells, should they become malignant. Thankfully, there are cells known as suppressor cells, which keep the body's cells from attacking its own. But if these suppressor cells are not functioning properly, the body's healthy cells can be attacked. The result is called auto-immune disease.

As you can see, the immune system is crucial because it seeks and destroys every uninvited invader that enters the body with murder on its mind. So it stands to reason that keeping your immune system in tip-top operating condition should be our number one priority.

The strength of the immune response to the invader is dependent upon the strength and condition of the host's immune system. If the immune response is inadequate, the invaders will not be destroyed. Instead they will multiply and invade the cells of the body.

If your immune system should quit functioning one day, you would be left with absolutely nothing to protect your body from viruses, bacteria and infections. That would be like playing Risk with no armies to protect your territories against invaders. As you can imagine, you would lose!

11

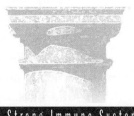

A Strong Immune System

ENEMY INFILTRATORS

As powerful and yet versatile as the immune system is, like any army, it is also susceptible to infiltrators that undermine its power and try to bring about its collapse. Of course, viruses and bacteria try to get in. But other infiltrators are more covert. If we can pinpoint these infiltrators, major or minor, we can work on eliminating them from our lives.

OUR POLLUTED ENVIRONMENT

ACCOMPANYING OUR TURBO lifestyles are the continual challenges that war against our immune system from the outside—the air we breathe, the water we drink and the food we eat. The population growth in America has caused a real health problem—overcrowded highways with thousands of trucks, cars and buses sending toxic fumes into the atmosphere and polluting the air you and I breathe. That's not to mention the smoke stacks from the industrial plants that permeate the air with millions of chemicals just ready to be inhaled.

Our cells are bombarded with toxins that are weakening our immune systems, causing respiratory infections, breathing problems and a host of other ailments. Our drinking water, with

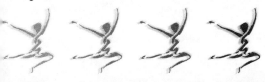

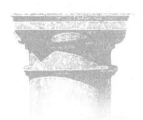

Symptoms like headaches, itching, rashes or fatigue can be signs of the beginning stages of an immune system breakdown.

all its chemicals, pollutants and bacteria, is another means by which invaders get into the body.

The pollutants have free radicals, which are impaired molecules that try to attach themselves to cells. The free radicals attach themselves to the good cells in our systems, and over time they break down cellular function. If our cells are continually challenged like this, they will weaken and allow disease and illness to have their way.

All these things weaken the immune system and can eventually cause it to break down. Symptoms like headaches, itching, rashes or fatigue can be signs of the beginning stages of an immune system breakdown. This constant assault of pollution on our immune system can eventually cause our superstructure to collapse.

Even the foods we eat can work against our immune systems. Most people will eat anything on their plate before carefully considering potential health risks that nitrites, nitrates, food additives, processed foods saturated with chemicals or rancid, oil-soaked fast food can have.

My approach to eating has changed over the years. Now I am convinced that eating foods compatible to one's blood type will save a lot of unnecessary trips to the doctor, lower healthcare costs and help us enjoy a more desirable lifestyle. Just as you and I have no control over the color of our eyes, neither do we have control over which foods are better for us biochemically than others. It's in our genes.

For example, if a blood type A person consumes dairy products, there's a good chance the result will be an overabundance of mucus in the respiratory system and the lining of the airway passages. This is due to the lectins found in those particular foods that are not compatible to the A blood type antigen. The subsequent mucus buildup then creates a breeding bed for infections and bacteria. Give the same dairy products to people with blood type B, and they will not experience any such reactions because those particular foods are compatible to their blood type antigen.

It is amazing to realize and appreciate how perfectly designed the blood type antigens are and how powerfully they work in the immune system.

The immune system successfully defends up to approximately 95 percent of the attacks of any uninvited intruders.[1] It's the remaining 5 percent of invaders that get into our bodies that cause all the diseases and illnesses. In consideration of this 5 percent, we should do all we can to protect this Pillar of Health.

Factor into that all the stressful events in our daily lives, our lack of dietary supplements and our lack of exercise or physical activities. Then ask yourself if there is not a remote chance of your health being challenged every day! That's why we should do all we can to fortify our immune systems.

HEALTH FACT BOX

Research is proving that there is increasing bacterial resistance to many antibiotics that once cured bacterial diseases readily. Due in part to the rise of resistance to antibiotics, the death rates for some communicable diseases (such as tuberculosis) have started to rise again.[2]

Seven Pillars of Health

ENDLESS PHARMECEUTICALS

THE EASIEST ROAD to take every time we get sick or experience some form of symptomatic reaction is to get a prescription for a medicine.

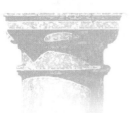

This line of thinking has been passed down from generation to generation, but there's a real problem with it.

God created the body with the precise ability to heal, detoxify and energize itself. Somewhere along the line we bought into the idea that it is easier to swallow a pill than to avoid what is causing the problem.

Somewhere along the line we bought into the idea that it is easier to swallow a pill than to avoid what is causing the problem.

In her book *Poisonous Prescriptions,* chemist Dr. Lisa Landymore-Lim states, "Given that a poison is ANY substance that when introduced into or absorbed by the body injures health or destroys life, most of today's pharmaceutical preparations, because of their harmful effects, may be labeled poisonous."[3] Dr. Landymore-Lim provides an insight into the poisoning nature of pharmaceutical drugs. Guess what the side effect of these medicines is? That's right—a challenged immune system.

Medicines have other side effects as well. Just read the insert from the pharmacy when you get your next prescription. I'm astounded by the fact that many people would never dream of reading the side effects of the medications that the doctor prescribes, but they will argue tooth and nail that taking vitamin C could be detrimental to one's health.

Not only are antibiotics often unnecessary, but they frequently destroy the helpful intestinal bacteria and deplete certain vitamins. A study by doctors at Cleveland's University Hospital has shown that even aspirin compromises the infection-fighting ability of the white blood cells.[4]

Enemy Infiltrators

People need to realize that although antibiotics may be necessary to treat certain bacterial infections, they can have detrimental effects on the body. They should be used only when absolutely necessary—not for viral infections. A doctor friend from Indianapolis confessed to me that throughout his medical training years, the primary thing he was taught was how to put bandages on the symptoms. The causes of the problems remained untreated.

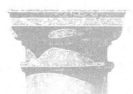

I am of the mind-set that it is my responsibility to do all I can from a natural perspective to prevent and maintain the health of my God-given body.

I am not bashing the medical community—I believe there is a place for conventional medicine. But my prayer is that some day the conventional medical community and the alternative medicine community will join hands and work together for the betterment of the American people. I am of the mind-set that it is my responsibility to do all I can from a natural perspective to prevent and maintain the health of my God-given body. If I have tried everything but have not succeeded, then I consider visiting the medical community.

Prevention, precaution and protection preserve our health. If you are trying to keep your immune system strong and healthy so it can keep you strong and healthy, avoid unnecessary medications and work on building your immune system.

Daily Stress

Due to our fast-paced society, all of us are exposed to lifestyles that are saturated with stress. Our bodies are living daily under stressful conditions, but I'm sure this is not news to you. You understand the stress of family life, raising children, spousal relationships—and, of course, the relatives. Then there is the stress in our occupations—the endless pressure from deadlines, sales meetings, appointments, bosses and coworkers.

Almost everyone experiences financial stress to some degree— the cost of living, insurance rates, gasoline prices, childcare, the economy. Many people have more days in the month than they have paycheck to cover the expenses.

Though stress is not a bug that infiltrates our immune system, it certainly affects it. Stress can weaken our immune system and keep it from operating efficiently, making us more susceptible to attacks from viruses and bacteria.

Pollution, drugs, stress—these infiltrators can weaken the immune system. Then, little problems can lead to bigger problems. Serious diseases are linked to immune system failure.

Autoimmune Disease

WHILE OUR MAGNIFICENTLY designed immune system is responsible for protecting our superstructure from sickness and disease, we have learned that it is continually being challenged by the pollutants in the air, water and soil plus all the drugs and medications we take.

Taking medications for too long of a period of time can cause the body to build up an immunity to the medication. With sleeping pills (not barbiturates), for instance, after taking them for a while, the body requires more of them to have the same effect. After years of being challenged by different medications, the immune system can turn on its own cells. The worst case scenario is that a person may contract an autoimmune disease.

Autoimmune diseases are simply the results of the immune system breaking down. It can no longer read the radar screen properly, and consequently it cannot distinguish friend from foe. The system then makes autoantibodies, which attack its own cells. They destroy their own organs and cause inflammatory responses. Some examples of autoimmune disease include amyotrophic lateral sclerosis (Lou Gehrig's disease), chronic fatigue syndrome (CFS), rheumatoid arthritis, AIDS and lupus.

CANCER

WITHIN EACH CELL is a code, generally referred to as DNA, that is duplicated over and over again as the cell reproduces. It is extremely important to protect this code in order for the cell to reproduce correctly. This protection is totally dependent upon the immune system. If a carcinogen, or cancer-causing agent, makes it past the immune system protectors and is allowed to disturb or distort the code and cause it to reproduce in an uncontrolled and erratic manner, then that cell becomes mutant. The result may well be the development of a malignant tumor and the beginning of cancer.

When the immune system detects the beginning of cancer, it begins its seek-and-destroy mission. The immune system works in two ways to fight cancer. If the carcinogens have not yet entered the cell, the immune system sends out the seek-and-destroy troops to stop them before they take hold. A healthy immune system will also work to destroy the mutant, cancerous cells that have already formed in the body. So if you can supercharge your immune system, it can defeat and in some cases reverse the cancer process.

The immune system is vital to the fight against cancer. With its help, the body can fight the battle against cancer—and in many instances, be victorious. Immunotherapy is a new way of treating cancer that uses our body's natural defense system, the immune system. It has been used successfully to treat several kinds of cancers, including skin and kidney cancers and some lymphomas. As more and more research is done, we will become better able to help our immune system win the battle against cancer.[5]

So, is there anything we can do to keep the immune system as healthy as possible? The good news is that we can definitely shore up our immune system and keep it working at top efficiency.

12

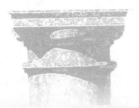

KEEPING THE IMMUNE ARMY
STRONG

If we truly understand the life-protecting function of our immune system and the seriousness of its potential breakdown, then we cannot help but be concerned about protecting it. Millions of people suffer from frequent colds, recurring bouts of the flu, headaches, migraines, hay fever, sinus infections and allergies—all obvious symptoms of a challenged immune system that is possibly losing its battle against the enemy invasion.

The body creates two hundred thousand new immune cells and thousands of antibodies every second in order to be strong enough to defend its superstructure. This means that millions of cells have to be rebuilt every day. It is absolutely necessary for our bodies to get the adequate nutrients essential for this day-to-day combat. It would behoove everyone who reaches for medications and drugs that mask the symptoms to reconsider their damaging effect on the immune system, then take the proper steps to naturally build the immune system instead.[1]

Many things help strengthen the immune system, including exercising, minimizing medication, avoiding hazardous environmental pollutants, lessening contact with radiation (x-rays included) and learning how to de-stress. Taking antioxidants also helps to eliminate free radicals from the system. But the one aid to strengthening the immune system that I believe is very important has to do with blood type.

Immune System Health Through the Blood Type Connection

ALL CELLS HAVE a chemical marker that is used by the immune system to determine whether the cell is friend or foe. These markers, referred to as *antigens,* are part of the cell's chemical make-up.

When various foreign bacterial, viral and parasitic antigens enter our bodies, the immune system responds by producing antibodies to destroy the intruding enemy antigens. It is the B cells in the immune system that produce these antibodies. When the T cells recognize the production of antibodies, they bind to the foreign antigens to help in the fight against these intruding antigens. The enemy antigens try to change or disguise their appear-

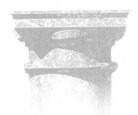

The antigens that determine your blood type are the most powerful in the body.

ance in order to evade capture and annihilation. Of course, the immune response is so accurate that the T cells and the antibodies simply glue themselves to the enemy antigen, clumping them together for easy disposal.

But some immune systems are friendlier to a particular enemy antigen than others. The immune army of people with blood type A, for instance, sometimes has a problem identifying certain invaders that have the same A-type antigen that the immune army has. That makes it more difficult to pick up the invader on the radar screen.

The blood type A system has to work to fight off the attack of foreign antigens with A-type antigens. As the immune system works to escort out the intruder, the person may get sick and have to fight the sickness. This same process would occur when another blood type person was fighting off foreign antigens that carried that same blood type antigens.

HEALTH**FACT**BOX

The antigens that determine your blood type are the most powerful in the body. When these different blood type antigens are functioning properly, they become the immune system's greatest army. Remember, the reproduction of most of the antibodies usually requires the presence of the invaders, either through a vaccination or an infection. But this is not the case with blood type antibodies. They are produced automatically by the body and are always available to do battle. This makes them invaluable.

Each blood type responds to invaders such as bacteria, virus or parasites in a uniquely different way. So it is important to be aware of your blood type to watch for certain immune system responses.

Specific associations exist between blood types and autoimmune disorders. Because of the association that blood type has with the immune system, it is normal to find that certain diseases are more common to certain blood types. The blood type O person is a predominant sufferer of arthritis, which is an autoimmune disease. That means the type O person must be aware of the responses that

112

take place when eating certain foods, such as white potatoes, which can induce inflammatory reactions in the joints.

Blood type A persons will often experience arthritis, but with puffiness, painfulness and debilitating breakdown of multiple joints. Blood type A persons can experience these responses to stress as well. In fact, they are known to be more high strung and may, therefore, innately bring on rheumatoid arthritis-like symptoms.

Multiple sclerosis and Lou Gehrig's Disease are more common to blood type Bs because of their tendency to contract slow-growing viral and neurological disorders. Some researchers believe that these two diseases are caused by a virus contracted at a young age that has B-like antigens. Since the immune system of blood type Bs cannot produce anti-B antibodies, these viruses can slowly develop over many years. This is a classic example of how the invader has fooled the immune response.

AB blood types are at high risk for these B-like diseases as well because their bodies do not produce anti-B antibodies either.

Immune System Health Through a Healthy Diet

By now I'm sure you agree that strengthening the immune system is a good idea. There are a number of ways by which we can do this. One of the ways to strengthen the immune system may be something you have not considered before. But I consider it to be extremely important. It is this: Since our cells have only what we put into our bodies to work with, the choices that we make about the foods we eat are critically important to our immune system.

Contrary to popular belief, even when we attempt to get proper nutrition by eating fresh, wholesome foods, it is impossible to receive the same abundance of nutrition from them today as people did over fifty years ago. Many of our parents and grandparents ate foods from their gardens or from the garden of the local vegetable seller. My father and his father grew their own vegetables, so their meals were prepared with fresh produce, grown from uncontaminated soil.

Unfortunately, it is not like that today. I remember listening a few years back to a lecturer talking about the condition of our air, water and soils. He gave a comparison of the nutrient value of a bowl of fresh spinach back in the forties vs. one today. His question for us was, "How many bowls of spinach would it take today to equal the nutrient level of that one bowl back in the forties?"

Some answered ten, others twenty. But he explained that because of the damage to the soils and water from chemicals, pesticides and fertilizers, it would take *seventy-five* bowls! Even if he was a little wide of the mark, that's still a tremendous difference!

IMMUNE SYSTEM HEALTH
THROUGH DIETARY SUPPLEMENTATION

THINGS JUST AREN'T the same as they were, so it behooves us to take precautionary measures to safeguard our health. When we take in consideration the fact that the average diet of the people in our society consists of fast foods and processed foods, it makes good sense that we enhance our nutrition with dietary supplements. The nutrients that are lost through depleted soils, improper food preparation, poor food choices, missed meals, sickness or stress can often be made up by dietary supplements.

A brilliant approach to enjoying a healthier life is to start with a complete colon-cleansing program. Regardless of how well we eat or exercise, we must take steps toward cleansing our invironment. Without periodic cleansing and scrubbing of the porous walls of the colon, we can acquire a mucous and fecal buildup that interferes with the proper absorption and assimilation of the foods and vitamins we are taking. After our colons are cleansed, we can take dietary supplements, knowing our bodies are getting the full value from them.

HEALTH **FACT** BOX

Keeping your lifestyle healthier is dependent upon a strong immune system. Listed below are only a few of the foods, spices and herbs that can play an important part in strengthening your immune system. The immune system of each blood type varies from the other and may have unique nutritional requirements.

Type A
Spices/herbs—Tamari, echinacea
Vegetables—Maitaki mushrooms, garlic
Soy
Beans/legumes—Lentils
Nuts/seeds—Peanuts and/or nut butter

Type B
Spices/herbs—Kelp, rose hips
Vegetables—Garlic, potatoes, cabbage, leafy greens and yams

Type AB
Spices/herbs—Kelp, echinacea
Vegetables—Garlic, potatoes
Soy
Beans/legumes—Lentils
Nuts/seeds—Peanuts and/or nut butter
(All compatible vegetables for type A and B are compatible for type AB except tomatoes. Type AB can enjoy them without any negative reactions.)

Type O
Spices/herbs—Kelp
Vegetables—Garlic, broccoli

You are unique, and your specific nutritional requirements may differ from mine. Some people require a specific combination of nutrients for their specific condition. Let me use the example of fibromyalgia because it seems to be common, especially in women, in this day and age.

Dietary supplementation for fibromyalgia

Fibromyalgia (FMS) for the most part is considered a rheumatic-like disorder characterized by chronic achy muscular pain with no obvious physical cause. It seems to affect most commonly the lower back, neck, shoulders, back of the head, upper chest and thighs. It is often difficult to pinpoint the exact area of pain, and it can affect almost any part of the body.

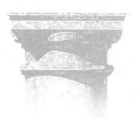

The nutrients that are lost through depleted soils, improper food preparation, poor food choices, missed meals, sickness or stress can often be made up by dietary supplements.

The most distinctive feature of fibromyalgia is what is known as the "trigger points," eighteen spots that have been identified by the ACR (American College of Rheumatology) as extremely tender to normal touch. To confirm a diagnosis of fibromyalgia, a patient must have tenderness at eleven or more of these trigger points.[2] The stiffness and pain that is usually described as throbbing or shooting, even stabbing, is greatest in the morning, but can occur throughout the day as well.

Symptoms that are experienced by fibromyalgia sufferers may range from chronic headaches, skin sensations and irritable bowel syndrome to anxiety, palpitations, memory impairment, dry eyes and mouth, irritable bladder, dizziness and impaired coordination. As the condition worsens, most sufferers are unable to perform daily tasks such as ironing, lifting or climbing stairs because of the day-to-day painfulness of their condition.

Fibromyalgia most commonly seems to be experienced by women, though men can suffer from it also. It strikes about 3.4 percent of American women and 0.5 percent of American men.[3] It appears that this condition starts in young adulthood and worsens as the individual ages. Though there is no real evidence of its cause, it seems to be related to the immune system.

The problem I have observed when working with fibromyalgia clients is that although they may have been struggling with the disorder for many years, the only treatment they have received from their doctors has been continual prescriptions for medications that never seemed to relieve their suffering.

While conducting several fitness classes for fibromyalgia sufferers, I heard their horror stories of being medicated by their physicians with everything from anti-inflammatory medication to antidepressants, sleeping pills and even morphine. Nearly all of them were overweight due in part to the lack of exercise, but also because of the reactions to the variety of medications. They often had lifeless eyes and appeared drugged. In fact, they were human medicine cabinets. Most said that after they had been treated (in some cases as long as twenty years), their physicians let them go and suggested they receive psychotherapy because they were hypochondriacs.

My own cousin, Melody, who lives in New York, had been suffering with fibromyalgia for ten to fifteen years. She was always tired and had terrible mood swings. Her condition became so bad that she had to leave her employment. Once she was diagnosed with FMS (years after she had the first symptoms), she started doing her own research to find help.

In February 1999 she contacted me, and I told her about a natural approach to beating FMS. I recommended that she first start with a colon-cleansing program to remove parasites, toxins

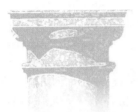

An ounce of prevention is worth a pound of cure. But maybe a pound of prevention is the cure!

from medications and bad bacteria and to clean her digestive system and help it get back in good operating order. I recommended an energy booster that works naturally to help balance her hormones. I suggested she drink a protein shake twice a day—one specific for her blood type. Plus, I gave her suggestions for changing her diet to foods that were compatible to her blood type. I also recommended aloe vera juice for stimulating her immune system.

Over one year later, my cousin told me, "I keep waiting for everything you suggested to stop working, but I keep getting better and better. I can't remember ever having a day where I could say I felt good. Now I have strings of days where I feel great!" She is happier and healthier than she has been for years.

I am in no way suggesting that you should not see your physician or that supplements should be taken in place of medical treatment. For anyone who is suffering from a constant loss of energy or continued pain, and who is not getting relief through regular medical channels, my advice is that the person consider natural alternatives. If people will take the preventative measure to take care of their health, the trips to the doctor's office can be cut back significantly. An ounce of prevention is worth a pound of cure. But maybe a pound of prevention is the cure!

Dietary supplementation for blood type

Some people, because of their condition or the demands on their health, might require more or less than others in both supplementation dosage and variety. I would recommend that you keep your supplementation plan as simple but as personally designed as possible.

HEALTH **FACT** BOX

BLOOD TYPE NUTRIENT SUPPLEMENTATION

Blood Type A
- Vitamin C, 240 mg.
- Vitamin E, 201 I.U.
- Hawthorn, 5 mg.
- Echinacea, 5 mg.

Blood Type B
- Magnesium, 60 mg.
- Iodine, 112 mcg.
- Bromelain, 100 mg.
- Quercetin, 10 mg.

Blood Type AB
- Folic acid, 200 mcg.
- Vitamin E, 201 I.U.
- Vitamin E, 201 I.U.
- Vitamin E, 201 I.U.
- Vitamin E, 201 I.U.
- Echinacea, 5 mg.

Blood Type O
- Licorice root, 5 mg.
- Bladder wrack, 37.5 mg.
- Niacin, 50 mg.
- Calcium, 125 mg.

People of all blood types should take a multivitamin and mineral supplement in addition to these nutrients.

Seven Pillars of Health

To help strengthen the immune system and the heart and to build the body to resist infections and cancer, supplementing is highly recommended. In an ideal world we would eat only those foods that are compatible for our blood type, exercise regularly and get eight hours of sleep a night. But that might not represent your real world. So what can you do to make your world healthy for you and your family?

Undisputedly, the answer is to add dietary supplements to your meals and snacks. This is a surefire way of providing the necessary nutrients for a healthy body. Since I am a firm believer in the links between blood type, diet and good health, I suggest a few nutrients that each blood type may need as supplements.

If you would like to receive more information about a basic dietary supplement program designed for your blood type, please refer to Appendix A.

STAYING ON THE DEFENSE

HEALTHY CELLS ARE imperative for keeping your immune system in tip-top operating condition. The immune system is the health protector of your superstructure and the major contributor to a longer and greater quality of life. There is not much hope for a healthy, vibrant and energetic life without giving constant attention to protecting and nourishing your cells with proper nutrients, exercise and foods that are compatible to your blood type.

As a boy I learned a great lesson from playing Risk. If I wanted to win the game, I had to learn the significance of building up a strong defensive army on each of the territories I owned. In doing so, I was able to defend and protect my territories from the enemies that came to take away what was mine.

By keeping this Pillar of Health—your immune system—strong, you will be ready to do battle and win when the ugly face of ill health pops up and tries to take your health away.

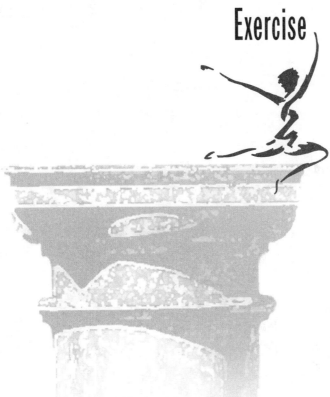

Exercise

If a man is lazy,
the rafters sag; if his hands are idle,
the house leaks.
—ECCLESIASTES 10:18

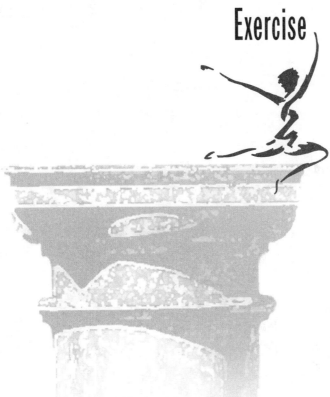

PILLAR FIVE

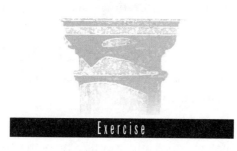

13

Exercise

THE BENEFITS OF EXERCISE

I t's impossible to hear the words *body* and *exercise* without thinking that we could be doing something about our flabby triceps or bulging bellies. Most people think of exercise as putting their bodies through sweaty, painful movements—an almost acceptable method of physical self-abuse—just for the reward of looking better. Beauty, looks, the body beautiful! Is that the only reward for exercising, or is there more?

It has now been shown that exercise or physical activity is more of a means for preserving and protecting our health than reducing waistlines. Medical reports, studies and research now support the fact that many health-related benefits accompany physical activity. In fact, the 1996 Surgeon General's Report on Physical Activity and Health says that inactivity is a serious nationwide problem.[1]

The new directives from the Surgeon General and the Secretary of Health and Human Services recommend that adults exercise moderately or engage in a physical activity for at least thirty minutes a day, which only 15 percent of American adults do. They also recommended that teens should engage in twenty minutes of vigorous activity three or more times per week. Secretary Donna Shalala went on to say:

> We had two important objectives in mind. We wanted to ensure that American not only added years to their lives, but added health to those years.[2]

The stronger the body, the better we are able to do everyday tasks, recreational activities and sports. The better shape our heart

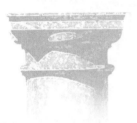

and lungs are in, the greater stamina we will have. Many people have difficulties performing simple tasks such as yard work or bowling because their bodies are not fit. In fact, they are unfit.

Some people have preexisting physical conditions that limit them from performing certain exercises or tasks. But even having an injured lower back or knee or other physical limitation is not necessarily a reason to avoid exercise completely. A smart approach to exercise will allow you to enjoy the benefits from exercise even if you are limited in what you can do.

It is now almost impossible to separate preventing illness from having a fit body. They are dependent on each other and are necessary elements of regular temple maintenance.

If you have physical limitations, consult with an exercise physiologist, a personal trainer or a health club that has competent instructors who can work with you to come up with exercises that will work for you.

Exercise is not limited to building biceps and reducing waistlines. It is a necessary part of one's lifestyle for the prevention of osteoporosis, heart disease, adult diabetes and problems associated with carrying extra weight. It is now almost impossible to separate preventing illness from having a fit body. They are dependent on each other and are necessary elements of regular temple maintenance.

The focus for incorporating regular exercise into your lifestyle should be twofold: improving your health through prevention of illness and maintaining a leaner, calorie-burning body.

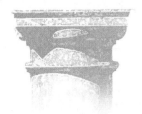

As you incorporate exercise into your life, remember that not everyone can be (or wants to be) a Mr. America or Miss America. Setting your sights on a realistic goal will save you a ton of frustration and disappointment, especially if your hope is to look like the model on the cover of *Cosmopolitan* or *GQ*. Let me tell you that "computerized cosmetics" have a lot to do with

Once you start exercising on a regular basis, your body will enjoy the wonderful physical stimulation it receives from it.

the flawless photos you see. Besides that, if the model you are trying to look like is five feet, eleven inches tall and you are five feet, three inches…well, you know the rest of the story.

Think for a minute of an old-fashioned slide rule. We want to slide away from the end of the scale that represents total abuse and neglect of our bodies while at the same time avoiding the opposite extreme of total obsession with our bodies. Our purpose is to find the happy medium that will give us satisfaction for the immediate but also protection and preservation of our health for the future.

Physical Benefits: A Healthy Superstructure

A NEW CLIENT once asked me what I did for my own personal training. After I told her how I trained and how often, she said in dismay, "You're going to have to keep that up the rest of your

HEALTH **FACT** BOX

Exercise does become a way of life—a wonderful way of life. Once you start exercising on a regular basis, your body will enjoy the wonderful physical stimulation it receives from it. Have you heard of "the pump"? That's the physiological response of your muscles' being gorged with blood after you exercise. It's such a healthy feeling—having your muscles tight and firm. And just like stirring up and getting rid of sediment in your gas tank, your body gets to release many of the toxins that have been stored up. You experience a fresh sense of well-being.

life!" I chuckled to myself because at the time I had already been training for nearly thirty years!

Exercise is not limited to attaining the body beautiful, even though that reason tops the list for most people. Exercise makes the human body healthier. As the individual participates in an exercise program, the body experiences an increase in core body heat, which in turn causes the body to eliminate toxins by sweating. Plus, exercise is the only means of flushing the lymphatic system, which means less of a chance of infection.

Exercise promotes circulation of blood throughout the entire body, delivering oxygen and nutrition to the cells and muscles, then dispelling carbon monoxide through heavy breathing. The lungs also get a thorough workout when a person exercises.

Through exercise, the musculoskeletal system is strengthened, including soft tissue-like ligaments and the tendons. The joints then get a break because stronger muscles do the work of holding the body.

As the overall physical condition of the individual improves, so does the body's resistance to injury, sickness and disease. Exercise stimulates the immune system, thereby contributing to building the body's defense mechanism against sickness, disease and fatigue. Regular exercise allows the body to utilize insulin properly and speeds the metabolism to burn calories more efficiently. All these contribute to a healthier body.

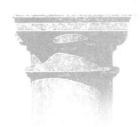

Your body was not designed to be sedentary; it was designed to be physically active.

After you start exercising regularly, when you miss a workout or two, you will notice that your body almost craves that stimulation. Your body was not designed to be sedentary; it was designed to be physically active. Your body will adjust to the stimuli you give it and will continue to improve as you increase the stimuli.

MENTAL BENEFITS: AN ATTITUDE ADJUSTMENT

> Those who cannot change their minds cannot change anything.
>
> —GEORGE BERNARD SHAW

There is a mental side to physical exercise. An exercise program that has any merit requires increased motivation and tenacity, which comes from mental conditioning.

The psychological forces that work against us are obvious, particularly after we have made the conscious and deliberate attempt to rise up in the morning before going to work and exercise! These forces rear their heads after a full day on the job when we are

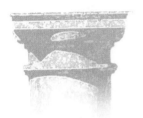

The "no" voice

is forever giving us the reasons

(excuses) why we should not or

cannot exercise.

driving to the gym. Mentally, we know we should go. But something is trying to interfere, even though we have already made a conscious mental commitment. How could this psychological opposition be taking place in our minds when we had already made plans?

I'll clue you in: Two opposing forces or mental voices are constantly vying for position in our psyches. One voice—the "no" voice—has been well developed, and we have learned to identify with it over our lifetimes. The other voice—the "yes" voice—is not as clear. Therefore we must take time to listen to it so we will be able to discern it.

The "no" voice

The "no" voice is forever giving us the reasons (excuses) why we should not or cannot exercise. This voice interrupts other areas of our lives as well, and in most cases it plays a huge role in preventing us from accomplishing our goals. This voice is influenced by the contacts it makes with the world around it—both positive and negative. The strength or volume of this voice comes from the subconscious memory bank, which has no ability to differentiate the information, only dictate it.

Let me give you an example to make this more clear. As your parents or caretakers guided you throughout the formative years of your life, you probably experienced a constant barrage of negative directives or negative reinforcement: "Don't touch that"; "Don't go near the TV"; "No, you can't go outside"—perhaps even some destructive "no" voices such as "You will never become anything in life"; "You're lazy"; "You're too fat"; "You're too short"; "You kids drive me crazy." Some of these were normal, healthy corrections a child must receive, and some were not. But all of them get stored in the subconscious mind or memory bank.

As your subconscious mind became filled with negative input, the "no" voice developed. Now, the "no" voice manifests itself outwardly by taking command of your decision-making process. This

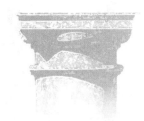

If you expose yourself to people and influences that are positive and helpful, you will enhance the development of the "yes" voice.

can cause you to back down from any challenging situation and prevent you from accomplishing your goals and doing the things you should.

This powerful voice is, in part, responsible for a vocabulary of negative words, such as "I can't...," "If...," "I doubt...," "I don't think...," "I don't have the time...," "Maybe...," "I'm afraid to..." or "I don't believe...." Your "no" voice is your enemy, and you must silence it.

The "yes" voice

The "yes" voice is the other, more subtle voice. It is slower in development, and both its vocabulary and volume need continual increasing. This voice always says, "Yes, go for it!"—no matter how challenging the situation is. As you can see, the "yes" voice is in a constant power struggle with the "no" voice. Once again, development of this voice can be enhanced by what is allowed to enter into the subconscious mind.

You did not have any choice about the information you received from your caretakers as a child, but you do have a choice now. You can dictate what you want to store in your subconscious mind. From which source, reference of information or influence

HEALTH FACT BOX

Remember, the subconscious mind does not judge what it receives as good or bad. It simply acts upon the information. So if you expose yourself to positive information, the subconscious will become filled with that. Then the "yes" voice will take control, and the negative enemy is defeated. When this happens, you will notice the change in your choice of words. Before you know it, you will hear yourself saying things like, "I can," "I will expect the best," "I know," "I will make time," "I am confident" and "I do believe."

will you choose to draw—positive or negative? Yes or no? By avoiding negative people or negative influences, you can block the power of the "no" voice. If you expose yourself to people and influences that are positive and helpful, you will enhance the development of the "yes" voice.

I once worked with a pageant contestant who was over-whelmed by some fears and challenges ahead. I encouraged her by asking her to remind herself of the following whenever she felt she needed it: "The bigger the problem, the smaller the God. The bigger the God, the smaller the problem."

When the "yes" voice has control, your view of the challenges in life becomes positive. The goals you set for yourself will be more rewarding because you will have done more than reached that goal; you will have learned how to make things happen!

The power struggle between these two voices will always be

present, but the one you choose to listen to will determine the outcome of your exercise program—and your life!

I'll let you in on something I've noticed over the last thirty years: I have never known anyone to leave a good workout saying that he or she should not have exercised! Afterward, people are always glad they did it.

Fill your environment and your life and your mind with positives, and learn to obey the "yes" voice!

Total Person Benefits: Well-Being

WHY DO PEOPLE choose to make exercise a consistent part of their lives? For myself as well as many other exercise keepers (those who *keep* exercise in their life), the answer is not the health benefits (though they are tremendous) but the positive inner experience associated with the exercise itself. When people reach this inner mind-set of enjoying the exercising itself—and many do reach that point—they become instinctive exercisers.

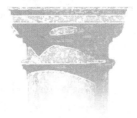

Certainly we all need to gain the health benefits as well as the shapelier bodies that come from exercising. These *external* benefits keep our motivation up. But if we

I have never known anyone to leave a good workout saying that he or she should not have exercised!

focus solely on them, we can lose the motivation that keeps us on track for the long haul. To become instinctive exercisers we must learn to enjoy the movement and the exercise itself. Learning to do so is imperative to move from sedentary living to a life of regular exercise.

One way to view exercise motivation is on a continuum from external benefits to internal benefits. External motivation places

HEALTH **FACT** BOX

MOTIVATING FACTORS OF EXERCISE

External benefits
- Exercise reduces the risk of disease.
- Weight management is easier with exercise.
- Exercise requires a disciplined mind.
- Exercise meets an expectation.

Internal benefits
- Exercise feels good.
- Exercise is enjoyable.
- Exercise satisfies my desire to keep fit.
- Exercise gives immediate gratification.

emphasis on doing a behavior for its rewards or outcomes, thereby focusing on the result. Internal motivation focuses on doing a behavior for its own sake.

Setting clear-cut goals is necessary to avoid distractions and to keep focused. If you have been bored before with exercising, most likely you became bored because you never developed clear, specific goals. It is impossible to get totally absorbed in your exercising if you do not know where you are going.

I have overheard people at the gym say that they were going to get on bikes and just pedal away. That often is a sign of someone who has not made clear-cut or precise goals, but is just wandering.

When I go to the gym, I am not the most sociable person there. That's because I am focusing on what I am doing. I have learned to develop a strong ability to concentrate during my workouts. When I perform a particular exercise, I mentally envision the muscle functioning. I actually see it contract and relax. In this way, I enjoy the movement and the exercise itself.

Because concentration can easily be disrupted in an open gym environment, you might try using a computerized machine at a health club because it is personalized and usually in a private room. Hiring a

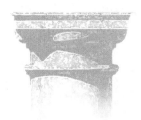

Internal motivation focuses on doing a behavior for its own sake.

personal trainer who understands your interests and goals can also help you to avoid distractions so you can get totally absorbed in the exercise.

Keep in mind that the reason for setting goals is to focus on the task at hand. For example, I can have different goals when I go for a walk. Some days my goal is to walk fast. Other days my goal is to slow it up and see what the neighbors are doing with their landscaping. The next day I might feel social, so I ask Lori to go with me. By varying my goals, my interest stays high, and I stay motivated.

I realize that many people conjure up enough will power to exercise, but they want to detach themselves from the exercise by reading or watching TV while doing it. In some cases, particularly for the beginner, a little disassociation can help a person do the exercise program. However, too much disassociation from the body during exercise lessens a person's awareness of the physical experience.

Ultimately the fitness journey will bring into balance the whole person—body, soul and spirit. The mental connection that is involved in the fitness journey will give control to the "yes" voice. Emotionally, people climb out of the dark valley of low self-esteem and negativity. *Because I've benefited and feel better, I will treat you better and encourage you. I can now be all that I can be. I like myself, so I can risk liking you.*

Seven Pillars of Health

As human beings, our make-up is tri-part: body, soul and spirit. Each is directly affected by the condition of the other. The ultimate goal is to create a balance for optimum physical, emotional and spiritual harmony. Exercise is one way to bring harmony to all three areas.

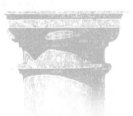

Finally, sharing all this positive emotional and psychological good with others will enhance your well-being. *I feel good, so I can be a good neighbor and a good friend. Because I have learned how to overcome the physical, mental and spiritual obstacles, I can challenge and encourage you to tap into your hidden resources.*

Real freedom comes from having boundaries, not being without them.

The first step to all these positive benefits to exercising is a new way to look at freedom.

FREEDOM TO FEEL AND BE YOUR BEST

FOR YEARS I have asked my clients their definition of freedom. Though their answers varied, the common denominator was being able to do whatever they wanted to do without any restrictions.

This definition of freedom is actually a form of bondage. Real freedom comes from *having boundaries,* not being without them. Let me explain.

Suppose for a moment that your goal is to lose weight. Can you imagine eating as much as you want, whenever you want, wherever you want, without any restrictions—and expecting positive results? That would be impossible. You would find that what you thought was freedom was not. As a matter of fact, the very mind-set that freedom means no boundaries has contributed

134

to the health problems many Americans are troubled with today.

Let me show you freedom from a different perspective. I'm sure you remember your mom saying, "This medicine might not taste good, but it's good for you," or "In life, there will be times when you have to do certain things that you don't want to do." Well, she was right. And she was talking about freedom.

HEALTH FACT BOX

The more you exercise, the more physical and mental energy you experience. The more often you exercise, the more endurance and muscular strength you develop. Everyday activities and tasks become easier. You enjoy the changes taking place in your body. You like what you see in the mirror. Your attitude is more positive, and your perspective toward other areas of your life is broadened.

Because you feel the physiological and physical improvements, you can't help but like yourself. You have disconnected the negative messages and now accept only the positive, so you have a whole new attitude that has lifted your self-esteem. You find yourself to be more assertive. All the giftedness and talent that has been suppressed for some time begins to surface. The people around you enjoy your company because of your positive outlook on life as well as your inspirational conversations and words of encouragement. Your spirituality is full of fruitfulness.

In a word, you have been freed—you are experiencing freedom

because of the boundaries you put on yourself to exercise whether you felt like it or not.

There is something to be said about the magnetism that exists in people who are physically fit. They naturally and automatically demonstrate commitment, discipline, balance and control. They exude good health and vitality. This discipline and balance naturally flows to the other areas of their lives, bringing harmony.

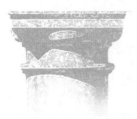

Freedom is the result you get when you are doing the things that you ought to be doing.

By listening to the "yes" voice, you will find it easier to exercise and enjoy the rewards of physical, mental and spiritual freedom that await you. What a powerful way to display spiritual fruits—through a well-kept temple. Freedom is the result you get when you are doing the things that you ought to be doing.

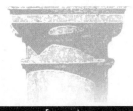

14

Exercise

How to Start Exercising

We are body, soul and spirit. Unfortunately, one of these areas is usually lagging behind the others, and often it is the body. The problem stems from lack of knowledge rather than laziness—even though laziness can be the culprit, too! Because the fitness world is plagued with fads, gimmicks and misinformation, the whole fitness journey can become frustrating, particularly if you are really interested in creating a better quality of life for you and your family.

Most people I watch in the gyms, spas and health clubs work diligently but unproductively because they lack exercise know-how. The proper tools are necessary to take your present physical condition to a level that is unimaginable. Remember: Knowledge is power. Even the Holy Scriptures say that God's people are destroyed from lack of knowledge (Hos. 4:6).

Once you understand and accept that physical fitness can contribute to providing you with a better quality of life, the only thing left is to be educated in exercise technique and what works best for you.

Let's start with some principles that will help you with your fitness journey.

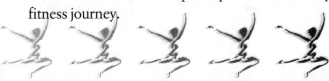

Seven Pillars of Health

Principle # 1: Exercise a minimum of three times weekly. If you exercise fewer than three days per week, you might find it difficult to lose body fat. On the other hand, you should start out slowly but progressively, allowing only what your fitness condition dictates. Too much too fast will cause potential injury and burnout, and will lead to dropout.

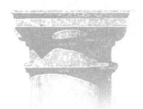

Get the kids away from the TV and the video games. Take them outside and play tennis or volleyball, take walks, throw the football around, play physical games or exercise together.

Principle # 2: Exercise for a minimum of fifteen minutes. Recent research has shown that as few as twelve minutes of exercise per session can produce cardiovascular improvement (but not much fat reduction). To assure more fat reduction, try aerobic training, which is low in intensity and long in duration. Then you will be able to exercise longer.

Principle #3: Warm up and cool down. Ideally, a ten- to fifteen-minute warmup of walking or cycling prepares the heart, lungs and muscles for a vigorous workout. It raises your core body temperature, which puts your body into a fat-burning mode. After your workout is over, it is a good idea to slow down the pace and cruise for about ten minutes or so. Stretching is a perfect way to cool down. This gives your internal machinery time to recover at an easy pace. Cool-downs also assist in eliminating much of the lactic acid buildup in the muscle tissue incurred in the main exercise time.

Principle #4: Drink 12 to 16 ounces of water about twenty minutes before each workout session. Then continue to drink water during the workout. It is important to rehydrate your system immediately after exercising, so make a few extra trips to

138

the water cooler then. The time to hydrate yourself is not when you feel thirsty, but throughout the activity.

Pay close attention to the environment around you. If you are exercising outdoors and it's hot and humid, you might be wise to go indoors or pass on the workout completely. Your body will have a difficult time cooling itself down in those conditions. Make sure you drink enough fluids throughout the day, every day.

Principle # 5: Practice safety during exercise. Monitor your heart rate throughout your workout sessions and stay within your ideal range. Remember to breathe. Sometimes people subconsciously hold their breath while exercising. If you do that, you won't last long. Plus, it can cause elevated blood pressure. Concentrate on exercise technique and form, not on the amount of repetitions left to do.

Principle # 6: Do a variety of exercises. Follow a baseline of exercises at least three times per week. But on the other days mix it up. Do some biking or hiking, go on walks or play some tennis or volleyball. Keep it interesting by varying your activities.

Principle # 7: Include family and friends. The nice thing about exercising is that it can be social. Some prefer to go it alone, but for the majority it is fun to share this positive experience. For couples who go for evening walks, exercise is a way to share being outside while sharing from the inside.

Learning about the physical condition of our young children today should motivate us to take them along with us. Their bodies need it, too. Parents must get involved in their children's lives and do physical activities with them. Get the kids away from the TV and the video games. Take them outside and play tennis or volleyball, take walks, throw the football around, play physical games or exercise together. Get creative so all the things you do are enjoyable for boys or girls. Their health is in your hands.

By the way, your program should have the simplicity and

HEALTH **FACT** BOX

SEVEN FITNESS PRINCIPLES

1. Exercise at least three times weekly.
2. Exercise at least 15 minutes.
3. Warm up and cool down.
4. Drink 12–16 ounces of water twenty minutes before you exercise.
5. Practice safety during exercise.
6. Do a variety of exercises.
7. Include family and friends.

flexibility to be conducted in the privacy of your home or at a health club, if you prefer. It need not require complicated or expensive equipment. Your program should also be a time saver. Most people do not have a lot of time to spare, so keep it short but effective. Then you will be able to stay motivated for the long haul.

THREE COMPONENTS OF AN EXERCISE PROGRAM

OBVIOUSLY, IT IS impossible for me to design a personal exercise program for everyone who reads this book. But I can give you an idea of what your body requires and what an exercise program should provide you.

All exercise programs should consist of the following three components:

Aerobic conditioning. Exercises that enhance the cardio-respiratory system—such as walking, jogging, cycling and stair-climbing—are aerobic conditioning. (This does not refer to aerobic high-impact classes.) Aerobic exercising is doing something that keeps your heart rate sustained at 60 to 70 percent of maximum

140

heart rate. (See Appendix B to calculate target heart rate.)

The benefits of aerobic conditioning include strengthening the heart and lungs, improving circulation, improving cholesterol ratings and lowering body fat percentages. When doing moderate intensity exercise such as aerobic conditioning, fat is the primary energy source used by the body for fuel. So this is a good fat-burning activity.

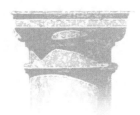

When doing moderate intensity exercise such as aerobic conditioning, fat is the primary energy source used by the body for fuel. So this is a good fat-burning activity.

Strength training. Exercises that enhance a muscle's ability to exert force against resistance produce strength. Isometric exercises, negative resistance training, floor or free-hand exercises and manual resistance exercises are good examples of strength training. Multistation exercise machines, conventional cables and pulleys with weight stacks, plate-loaded equipment and handy free weights such as barbells or dumbbells are all tools of the trade for strength training.

Strength training shapes and tones muscles as well as making them stronger. Strength training will help elevate your good cholesterol (HDL) levels, which in turn contributes to lowering the bad cholesterol (LDL). Strength training stimulates your metabolic rate for burning fat calories. Strength training also aids in the prevention of injury by promoting proper balance among the various muscle groups.

Flexibility training. This type of training enhances and promotes the ability to move a joint through the full range of motion (ROM) without discomfort. Full range of motion for every joint is a must for proper joint action.

HEALTH**FACT**BOX

THREE COMPONENTS
OF AN EXERCISE PROGRAM

1. Aerobic conditioning
2. Strength training
3. Flexibility training

Static stretching is a form of stretching that gently promotes elongation and flexibility of muscle and soft tissue. Stretch the muscle until it becomes comfortably tight but not painfully tight. Then hold that position for approximately fifteen to thirty seconds. Release the stretch and take the muscle back to its original position.

This form of stretching does not involve any ballistic or bouncing motion. Do not jerk the limbs you are stretching, but simply apply a constant, gentle stretch. Be careful not to stretch beyond that comfort point, or you will not be able to relax the muscle; therefore, you will not benefit from the stretching exercise. Repeat this procedure four to six times per muscle group as well as every time you feel the need to stretch.

The benefits from stretching and flexibility exercises are a decrease in muscle and joint injury and soreness and the lengthening of muscle and connective tissue. Stretching will reduce stress and increase your ability to relax.

For years we have been taught to stretch before starting a strength training session, power walk or run. But I would prefer to see people warm up the muscles first, then stretch them out. For

HEALTH FACT BOX

What are your goals? Perhaps you want to redesign your body or strengthen it for a specific sport or activity. Or maybe you just want to stay healthy. Whatever your goals are, they should be concise, short-term and obtainable. By setting short-term goals, you will have success.

example, the next time you decide to jog or power walk, it would be wise to walk gently for about ten minutes. Warm up those muscles by getting some blood pumping into them and some sinew fluid flowing in those joints. Then, after the short warm-up session, take time to stretch the muscles involved in your workout for that session.

Properly stretched muscles will perform at their optimum. Golfing, bowling, tennis, hiking, dancing, chasing the kids around—everything will become easier when your muscles are flexible.

SETTING FITNESS GOALS

EVERY TIME I do a seminar or workshop on exercise, I spend time afterward with a few people who are very intense about getting back in shape. The problem is that most of them want to make a quantum leap from their current condition (one that took twenty years of abuse or neglect to produce) to their goal. It would be nice if we didn't have to climb a ladder one rung at a time to get to the top, but that is the safest and surest way.

HEALTH**FACT**BOX

Many people like to measure their success by using their scale, but I prefer not to. The scale can only tell you how much gravity is pulling you down at the moment; it doesn't tell you the composition or quality of your weight. My suggestion is to throw out the scale and use one of the other measurements of success instead.

Part of climbing that ladder is having goals. Over the years I have observed that people who decide to make physical fitness a part of their lifestyle start with one or two basic goals in mind.

Exercise and healthy eating should become a part of your lifestyle, not a quick-fix. So set lifestyle goals. It is more likely that you will reach your goals by chipping away at them rather than trying to swallow them in one big gulp. Therefore, in my recommendations to a person in regard to eating, I always suggest that a person first use my 80/20 plan. If people can eat foods that are best for their blood type 80 percent of the time, they will be healthier and happier. The same goes for exercising. Instead of trying to max out on every exercise you do in the gym, try building up slowly week by week until you reach the goal.

If your goal is to lose four dress sizes, then set out to drop the first one. After you have reached that goal, go on to the next dress size. This will allow you to stay motivated because your short-range goals are being reached.

If your goal is to build more muscle on your chest, you will be most apt to succeed if you make your goal to gain the first inch.

Then set out for the next inch. This will establish a good foundation for success.

Create a way to measure your performance when setting goals. Let's say that you and your friend are taking walks every morning. You both walk three miles in sixty minutes and then call it quits. To measure your performance, set out weekly to increase your time. Thirty days later, you and your friend are finishing the same three miles in forty-five minutes. Your performance can be measured by the decrease in time it takes for you to walk those three miles. That decrease in time indicates an increase in fitness. (For a walking chart to measure performance, see Appendix C.)

In case you find yourself backsliding, a quick glimpse at your journal will help you get back on track.

Measuring your performance will provide the evidence of work being accomplished and will give you a means to evaluate your program. Remember, remaining motivated is the key.

TOOLS FOR MOTIVATION AND SUCCESS

I HAVE DISCOVERED several tools that have helped to keep this Exercise Pillar strong.

A fitness journal can monitor your fitness journey. It is always a good idea to write down where you are throughout your process. As you successfully reach your goals, you will have a record of what you accomplished. In case you find yourself backsliding, a quick glimpse at your journal will help you get back on track. An example of a journal page can be found in Appendix E. You can make copies as needed.

Write down your goals along with the method you have chosen

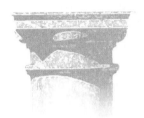

By having someone keep you accountable, you will put forth your best effort and stay committed. That person will become the one who gives you the compliments and encouragement that will help you stay focused.

of measuring your success. Include feedback and the rewards. Reviewing them from time to time will reinforce your strategy and your motivation.

Remember, some people enjoy using journals as a tool; others don't. I recommend them in the beginning to help you get started and stay on track. Later you may not need one to remain on track. Then you will instinctively know when to push yourself more.

Body fat testing and retesting have proven to be very helpful tools for monitoring success and providing evidence that you are accomplishing your goal. There are a few ways of having your body fat tested. One is with the use of calipers, which are instruments used by a personal trainer, exercise physiologist or specially trained person to take a reading of the thickness of your skin folds at various sites on your body.

Another method of testing body fat is an impedance machine that measures the resistance or time an electrical signal takes to travel through the body. This machine prints out the data that shows your body fat percentage and weight, your muscle weight and the percentage of water in the tissue.

These are safe, pain-free and harmless, and can be performed at your local YMCA or health club. Chart these measurements so you can follow your progress on a regular basis.

Feedback is most helpful when trying to stay focused on your goals. How many times has just a single word of positive affirmation been just the push you needed to continue? I love to see the glowing expression on the face of a person who is telling about the

HEALTH FACT BOX

TOOLS FOR EXERCISE SUCCESS

1. A fitness journal
2. Body fat testing and retesting
3. Feedback
4. Rewards

workers at the office commenting on how good he or she looked. There is nothing like a shot in the arm when you're wavering.

Generally, when you participate in an exercise class, hire a personal trainer or simply begin a program at home, people in your immediate life can help you stay accountable. A student of mine once said that hiring me as her personal trainer made her so accountable that every time she went out to dinner, she would see my face in her dinner plate!

By having someone keep you accountable, you will put forth your best effort and stay committed. That person will become the one who gives you the compliments and encouragement that will help you stay focused. As you stay focused and committed, and you keep giving it your best effort, others who see you will say positive things about you as well.

Besides the compliments from others, the positive way you feel about yourself and the progress you see will be wonderful feedback for you.

Rewards await you as you press on to success. Your reward could be getting into some of those beautiful clothes that you haven't been able to wear for months or maybe a shopping spree to purchase an entirely new wardrobe. Every time you reach an intermediate or short-term goal, consider rewarding yourself. Don't worry; you won't spoil yourself. But getting rewards every month can certainly help you stay committed.

Finally, the level of your success will depend solely on the level of your commitment. Making time for regular exercising is demanding and will challenge your integrity. Remember, you paid the price to get into the shape you're in now, so realize that you will have to pay your dues to get into the best shape of your life.

You have to admit, every time you see those joggers on the side of road or hear people talking about how healthy they feel since they made a commitment to exercise, you think you should be doing the same thing. Your body is a walking billboard—it publicly advertises what is happening in you. Your level of commitment to yourself and your program will not only benefit you physically, but mentally and spiritually as well.

From the start of your fitness journey, remember that you are in a constant state of transition. You will have some hurdles to jump. There will be times when you won't see any progress, you won't get any compliments, and you'll feel like quitting because you think you'll never reach your goals. When any negative thoughts come in, just remember that you are in a state of transition. You're not there yet, but you're getting there. Keep the momentum going.

15

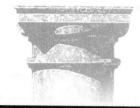

Exercise

Exercise and Body Redesigning

When you see an infomercial on television that shows a couple of fitness models demonstrating a piece of exercise equipment, you receive the message to get your body into great shape. Body shaping or redesigning can definitely be a benefit of exercise, but it requires consideration of body type, blood type, genetics, health issues and physical limitations.

Body Types

How is it that someone you know (and we all do know a person like this) can eat anything he or she desires and never put on a pound? Then there are people like us—we simply look at food and our pants tighten up. By understanding how genetic factors play a huge role in the success of your fitness efforts, you will be less likely to get discouraged and give up. Through proper application of the right exercise methodology for your genetics, you will experience greater success with less pressure and guilt, and you will reach your genetic potential.

It is estimated that 75 percent of our body typing comes

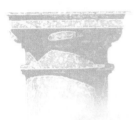

Heredity is not totally responsible for our shapes, because each one of us can do things to improve the not-so-perfect body we have been given.

straight from our genes. So the pressure is on your parents and their parents and their parents—not you! Heredity is not totally responsible for our shapes, because each one of us can do things to improve the not-so-perfect body we have been given.

If there is a true category of body types (and the jury is still out on this one), the question is, What am I working with? What are my bodily attributes? What works best for my body type?

Perhaps you have an apple-shaped body, with most of your weight in your upper body. To create a balanced physique, you would have to build up your lower body—the legs. But if you have a pear-shaped body, with most of the weight in the hips and thighs, you would not want to perform those bulk-building lower body exercises. Instead, you would do exercises that would fill out your upper body. However, if you have a banana-shaped body, then adding curves to your body will work best. The body type with which you were born must be factored into your fitness program if you want to have specific results.

Before I go any further, I want to make sure you understand that when I am talking about redesigning the body, I am referring exclusively to the physical body. Far too often people confuse their physical condition or appearance with the person on the inside! Remember, the body is only the compartment that houses the real you.

BODY TYPES AND EXERCISE

BEFORE I LIST the body types, their characteristics and exercise

Exercise and Body Redesigning

prescriptions, I must remind you that it is impossible to restructure your musculoskeletal system. In other words, if you have short clavicles (the bones that give your shoulders their width), but you desire wide shoulders, forget about it. If your hip bone measures thirty-five inches and you want thirty-inch hips, it's not going to happen. These are predisposed genetic traits that make up your body.

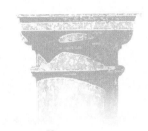

You cannot outsmart your genes, but you can use exercise strategies that are compatible with them.

But don't close the book yet. There is still hope! Through exercise, you can take your body's genetically given structure to a level of a shapeliness and new curves that did not come with the package. You cannot outsmart your genes, but you can use exercise strategies that are compatible with them.

These textbook body types may not describe you perfectly. As you examine yourself and your family members, you might discover that there is a little of each morph in your shape and size. But your body probably tends to have more characteristics of one over the others.

So, let's begin with the most traditional categories of body classifications. Is your body type an endomorph, an ectomorph or a mesomorph?

The endomorph

Endomorphs are people with bulky bodies. If your body type is an endo, then your main concentration should be losing body fat. Cardiovascular training works best for you. You should spend about 70 percent of your training time doing aerobic sessions. Up to 30 percent of your time should be in strength training. For the rest, do some form of stretching or flexibility training.

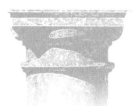

As you develop more muscle or lean weight, your body becomes more of a calorie burner because the body requires more energy (calories) to move muscle.

Aerobic training. Stay away from group fitness classes that conduct high-impact aerobics. Stay with low-impact exercises such as walking on the treadmill or riding a stationary bike.

Strength training. Concentrate on the large muscle groups (chest, back, arms, shoulders and legs) and keep the repetitions high and the weights moderate.

Flexibility training. Center your focus on stretching classes to strengthen the hips and the knees.

The ectomorph

The etco is the thinnest of all the body shapes. Ectos come with a stingy genetic disposition that fights against weight gain. For some it's a blessing; for others it's a curse. If this is your type, then special attention should be given not to overtrain. This body type will easily tap into its cellular reserves for muscle growth, repair or energy if the workout is too intense.

My recommendation is to spend approximately 80 percent of training sessions on muscle stimulation through strength training. Spend about 10 percent on cardiovascular training and 10 percent on stretching and flexibility training.

Aerobic training. Keep it to a minimum. Try stationary biking or using a treadmill, an eclipse or any preferred cardio workout. Keep the time between ten to twelve minutes. The best time for this is after your workout or on your off days.

Strength training. Every ecto should place most of the focus on strength training. To properly train, the ecto should use the heaviest weights possible for every exercise, while keeping the repetitions down to six or eight.

Exercise and Body Redesigning

Ideally, ectos, with their fast metabolism, need only to take each exercise to positive failure in order to stimulate their muscles to grow. In a pushing-type exercise, the pushing away of the weight from the body is the positive side, and the lowering or returning of the weight is the negative side. *Positive failure* occurs when an exercise cannot go any further than the last rep in the positive side of the exercise. Ectos should use a weight that will not allow them to go past six or eight reps, not even by one rep. That means using as much weight as possible. Keep the sets at three to four. Train one body part every five to six days.

Flexibility training. Concentrate on the major muscle groups—the lower and upper back, shoulders, arms, quadriceps (frontal thigh muscles) and hamstrings (rear thigh muscles). This is important for strengthening the joints.

HEALTH FACT BOX

All three body types are in need of aerobic training to help metabolize fat. But that training is not going to be enough to maximize fat burning. You should include strength training or redesigning in addition to your aerobic training for two reasons:

1. As you develop more muscle or lean weight, your body becomes more of a calorie burner because the body requires more energy (calories) to move muscle.
2. Strength training, by developing new muscle, actually reshapes your body and alters your appearance.

The mesomorph

If you are a meso, then genetically speaking you have been blessed with the ideal body type. Mesos have a naturally well-balanced, symmetrical physique and therefore can focus on their goals instead of concentrating on exercises that make up for their body type. Mesos respond very well to any exercise. They have a natural ability to build muscle weight easily with symmetrical balance.

Aerobic training and strength training. Split your training up between these two.

Flexibility training. Stretch the major muscle groups. Flexibility is necessary for joint strength.

Along with information for the body morphs just described, try incorporating the body shape guidelines below. Use them as a starting point, but experiment until you find what fits you best.

BODY SHAPES

FOR YEARS PHYSIOLOGISTS have used the apple and pear metaphors to help classify body shapes. Males are usually the classic apple shape, notorious for gaining weight around their upper torsos and mid-sections. Females are generally pear-shaped, storing most of their excess body fat on their thighs and hips. But my thirty-plus years of observation have proven that women in particular are typed as being either a pear, an apple or a banana.

The easiest way to determine your body type is by answering the following question: If I gain weight, where does most of it go?

- If you answer hips, thighs and buttocks, you are a pear.
- If you answer stomach, arms and back, you are an apple.
- If you answer both upper and lower, you are a banana.

When I was involved in the pageant industry, helping the women prepare for the swimsuit competition, I saw amazing and dramatic results from exercise. The majority of the female body types I worked with were the true pear shape. I recall one girl in particular who had very large hips, thighs and buttocks, a small waist, a flat bust line and narrow shoulders.

At the end of ninety days she had dropped five inches off her thighs, hips and buttocks areas. She had also added two inches to her bust measurement and her shoulder measurement. Her figure had gained the most pleasing symmetry that her body type would allow. Her body went from the genetic pear-shaped figure of 34-25-41 to a redesigned symmetrical 36-24-36.

Of course, her motivation and commitment level were extremely strong because of the competition. But this level of commitment is common once people identify their genetic structure and apply the proper exercise methodology.

We always want to place more emphasis on the weaker areas to bring them up to par with the stronger ones. This altering of your appearance will not change your genetic baseline, but it will bring out your genetic potential.

Remember, let your fitness condition—not the program—dictate how much exercise to do. If you are unfit, then start slowly and work up to the optimum exercises.

Apples

Aerobic sessions. Try treadmill, stair-climbing or cycling. These sessions should be short in duration and high in intensity. Build up to thirty minutes at about 65 percent of your maximum heart rate. Of course, this must be adjusted to your present physical fitness condition.

Cardiovascular interval training sessions. During a twenty- to twenty-five-minute workout, vary the intensity every few minutes. Exercise at 65 percent of your maximum heart rate for five minutes, then drop down to 60 percent again for the next five minutes. Continue varying your intensity for the whole workout.

Strength training (redesigning). Concentrate on the upper torso, specifically on your shoulders, chest and upper back. Keep the repetitions between ten and twelve, and perform three sets per exercise per body part. Start off at twenty to twenty-five minutes per workout.

Since you are heavy on the top and taper down at the hips and thighs, you should concentrate on heavy lower body exercises. Try incorporating squats, leg presses and calf raises. Do upper body exercises just for firming and toning the abs and pectorals.

Pears

Aerobic sessions. Try walking, cycling or treadmill. Your aerobic training sessions are nearly opposite to those for your fruitful friend, the apple. The intensity level is low, which means you can train for a longer duration. Aerobic training done for a long period of time will help metabolize fat storage. The length of your aerobic session is an individual thing, but go for a minimum of thirty minutes. You can work up to forty-five minutes or sixty minutes if you are advanced and want to make significant improvements. Anything longer is not as productive.

Cardiovascular interval training sessions. During a twenty- to thirty-minute workout, vary the intensity every few minutes. Exercise at 65 percent of your maximum heart rate for five minutes, then drop down to 60 percent again for the next five minutes. Continue varying your intensity for the whole workout. This will speed up your metabolism.

Strength training (redesigning). Focus on the chest, shoulders and arms. The repetitions should be eight to ten per set, with three sets per exercise per body part. This session should last up to twenty-five minutes.

Since your body is heavy at the hips, thighs and buttocks, then avoid completely any exercises that will bulk the muscles in the lower body. This includes any compound movements such as leg presses, squats or power deadlifts. Also avoid the stair-climbing

Exercise and Body Redesigning

machines and high-resistance stationary bike riding. Try isolation movements like high-rep 90-degree side leg lifts (hydrants) and iso-lunges. A hips isolation machine is excellent for targeting the hips and buttocks area. Also ride a stationary bike at low resistance.

Bananas

Aerobic sessions. Try walking, stair-climbing or cycling. You will want to keep the intensity low, allowing for a longer session. This aerobic session is done on your "off" days from your body redesigning workouts. Ideally, you should exercise from thirty minutes and build up to forty-five minutes. This will assist your body in losing excess body fat.

Cardiovascular interval training sessions. During a twenty- to twenty-five-minute workout, vary the intensity every few minutes. Keeping the intensity from dropping too low is best. But exercising at 65 percent of your maximum heart rate for five minutes or so and then dropping down to 60 percent for five more is a good mix. You will want to stimulate your metabolism.

Strength training (redesigning). Because your genetics typically lack curves, building muscle (lean not bulky) on the upper and lower body work best. Focus equally on the upper and lower body with compound exercises for the lower body such as bench squats, deep-knee bends or weighted lunges, and weighted exercises for the upper body such as dumbell chest press, around-the-world for shoulders and tricep/bicep dumbell exercises. Of

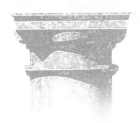

The most important exercise you will do in your fitness journey is taking the first step.

course, as with all body types, you will want to include abdominal exercises such as reverse crunches, twists and regular crunches. This session should go for twenty to twenty-five minutes.

Seven Pillars of Health

Since your body type is such that your upper and lower body are equal or straight up and down, then you are not as concerned with balancing your body's shape as you are to adding curves. By placing emphasis on reducing the waistline, broadening the shoulders and adding curves to your hips, this can be accomplished.

Taking the First Step of Faith

The most important exercise you will do in your fitness journey is taking the first step. As you move forward to fortify this Pillar of Health, you will discover that many more rewards await you. But the time to start is now. The more time you waste getting started on an exercise program, the longer you delay your rewards.

Practice keeping your eyes focused on your goal. Getting into the best shape of your life does not involve simply flipping through some high-fashion magazine and following a model's routine. Your body transformation will require a plan, the proper tools and a better understanding of your genetics, your shape and your motivation.

Give equal attention to all three parts of you—body, soul and spirit. Your body, the temple that houses your spirit, must be maintained with proper exercise and nutrition. Your soul, which sorts out your emotions, feelings and decision-making, needs to listen to your "yes" voice. And your spirit, which is in need of supernatural regeneration for everlasting life, can govern every relationship that comes across your path with unconditional love.

The rewards for committing to your fitness journey will lose some of their significance if they stop with you alone. Spread the good news of physical fitness. Turn your personal rewards into gifts of encouragement and inspiration for the people you meet along the way. Then your greatest reward will be the positive impact you make on the lives of others throughout your journey.

Remember, your body is a temple that holds something of great value—you! Taking care of it deserves your very best effort..

6

Rest and Relaxation

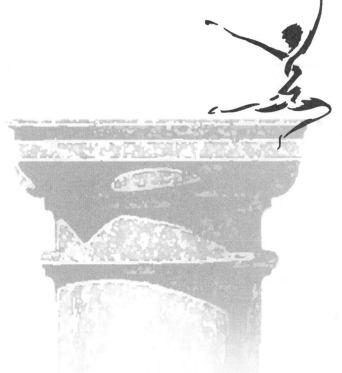

The sleep of a laborer is sweet.
—ECCLESIASTES 5:12

PILLAR SIX

16

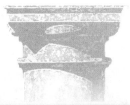

THE IMPORTANCE
OF R AND R

Lori and I were married in front of a waterfall at a resort in Jamaica. Then we stayed at this paradise, tucked away on the side of a mountain, for the most relaxing two weeks of my life.

Engulfed in tropical plants and flowers and abundant natural waterfalls and streams, we spent most of the time lounging around the heart-shaped pool and listening to the steel drums of the Caribbean band. Sometimes, we floated on rafts and let the sight of the tall, swaying palm trees put us to sleep.

But the most restful spot on the entire resort was right near our condo. I spotted it one day while walking over a little wooden bridge. There it was—a hammock stretched between two trees right next to the stream.

Eagerly, I slipped into it. The hypnotic sounds of water trickling over the rocks and birds chirping in the trees together with the steady swaying of the hammock put me right to sleep. The time I spent in that hammock really revived my overworked body and mind.

Whenever I think of rest and relaxation, those two blissful weeks of romance and nature come to mind.

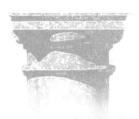

God gave us a model to go by: Rest! Take time to relax!

We all like the idea of resting and relaxing. But do we know their value? We are so overcharged and revved up all the time that the very idea of leaving all our deadlines for a three-day R and R weekend can make us crazy!

Yet even God took the seventh day to rest. I'm not sure He was actually fatigued or burned out from the preceding six days of creating the world. Nevertheless, God gave us a model to go by: Rest! Take time to relax!

Relaxing Body, Mind and Spirit

Rest is needed by our bodies to recover from physical stressors or even work, exercising, recreational activities and everyday tasks. Our minds need rest from emotional stressors too, such as family situations, marriage relationships, financial woes and employment or business concerns.

Rest and relaxation are absolutely necessary for spiritual rejuvenation. How long has it been since you got away by yourself and spent time recharging your spiritual batteries? Maybe this is what God also had in mind when He showed us that rest is an integral part of everyday life. Spiritual checkups are advisable on a regular basis.

The Overload Zone

Most of us today live with so much stress and busyness that it often takes a major jolt to get our attention. If you have reached the point where life is no fun anymore, then you just might be held hostage to the Overload Zone.

You end up in the Overload Zone when you get totally drained emotionally, physically and spiritually. Once you hit the Overload

HEALTH **FACT** BOX

ARE YOU IN THE OVERLOAD ZONE?

- Are you too busy to spend quality time with your spouse?
- Are you too preoccupied to fine-tune your marriage relationship?
- Do you spend little or no time with your children and/or teenagers?
- Do you lack spiritual stamina?
- Have you abandoned your quiet time of prayer and meditation with God?
- Are you less kind and friendly to others around you?
- Do you lack sensible, healthy eating habits?
- Is there no room left in your daily schedule for regular exercise?
- Do you always make excuses for not exercising?
- Do you feel run down and fatigued?

Zone, your work performance suffers. Your family life becomes more like a second job than a haven from the outside world, and your spiritual life and relationship with God become dead.

Before it is too late, take a minute or two to see if you can identify with any of the Overload Zone symptoms. If you identified with one to three of these symptoms, you need some fine-tuning. If you identify with four to six of them, you need a minor overhaul. If seven or more sounded too familiar to you, a major overhaul is the only thing that will save your downhill slide.

Seven Pillars of Health

Stop right now! Take a break! Make immediate plans for rest and relaxation, then address each area with which you identified. I'll show you how.

STRESS—THE MODERN EPIDEMIC

IF YOU SCORED high on the Overload Zone questions, then you need to de-stress. An overworked brain and an unused heart are typical red flags for stress. Progressive relaxation, a combined form of physical and emotional de-stressing, can help the brain and heart gradually return to their natural rhythms.

Think about it for a minute. How long has it been since you took a step back from your maddening pace to determine if your brain is overworked? Spending a few hours doing research on the information highway will show you how easy it is to become mentally stressed. Because of the overwhelming amount of information available to us today, we can easily become brain-tired without realizing it.

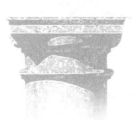

If you think you don't have time for eustress, then let me remind you that it is much easier to maintain your health than to try to repair it.

During any given day we find ourselves confronted with various forms of stress. If you live in this modern world, I hardly need to name them for you. Traffic, relationships, poor health, finances—these and more are responsible for anxiety in our lives.

Hans Seyle, often called the father of stress studies, is a pioneer in stress research. The kinds of stress I named in the previous paragraph are negative stress, which he calls *distress.* He calls positive stress *eustress,* or good stress.[1]

By adding eustress, or good stress, into our lives on a daily basis, we can become more balanced in our lives. Adding a thirty-minute

HEALTH **FACT** BOX

DE-STRESSING

The three stages of de-stressing:
- Identify the stress.
- Examine the stress to determine the root.
- Develop a stress management program that includes:
  - Alternative creative solutions to deal with the stress
  - Action steps you will take to manage the stress
  - A way to record your progress

workout followed by some form of stretching to your schedule would be adding good stress. Having a full body massage is another form of eustress. Even laughing and saying positive and complimentary things about others are forms of good stress.

Creating harmony in our body, soul and spirit is directly linked to the way in which we learn how to balance the distress and the eustress in our lives. Unfortunately, living in a fast-paced society keeps us striving for that balance.

If you think you don't have time for eustress, then let me remind you that it is much easier to maintain your health than to try to repair it. All the money in the world can never buy good health and a sound mind. If you are thinking to yourself that you don't have the time to de-stress, that in and of itself says that you need to. I'm sure you've heard the line, "You can pay me now or you can pay me later, but you are gonna pay me." That's exactly what happens with stress.

Less negative stress in our lives would be wonderful, but in a world as fast-paced as ours, that is only part of the solution. *The attitude we have toward stressful events is the important thing.* Someone once said, "Life is 10 percent how we make it, 90 percent how we take it." In and of itself, stress is not the problem; our perception of the situation is the bad guy. One man's dreaded family reunion is another man's picnic. We can deliberately change our way of thinking about a stressful situation so that its negative effect on us is reduced. It takes a little effort, but it will be worth it.

Perhaps you arrive home from work stressed from not only the workload, but also from office politics, pettiness and unfairness. If there is a person at home to talk with about your day, then you can get things off your chest. After a while, you will feel calmer. Perhaps you can even laugh at some of the things that made you uptight during the day. You remember together that life doesn't always run smoothly.

Once mentally relieved by the talk, it's a good idea to do something to de-stress physically, too. Perhaps taking a walk or enjoying a soak in the tub will help to bring down your blood pressure and heart rate.

Once you start noticing when you are stressed, take the measures that work for you personally to remove the stress from your life.

A first step in de-stressing our lives is identifying the source or sources of stress in our lives. What causes you the most stress? A person at work? Your boss? Your children's friends? Your lack of finances? Perhaps it's your health or a bad habit you have. Or maybe it's the health of a loved one.

Then, examine the stress to determine the root cause. Is it emotional, mental or physical? Why is this event particularly stressful for you? Maybe you have an emotional wound in a certain area that is pricked by the person at the office or by your boss. Perhaps you fear failing financially because that happened to your parents, and you lived through it. Or maybe it's just a character flaw you need to accept that you have and deal with, such as a bad temper or a sharp tongue. Understanding the root of the stress will aid you in changing your perspective toward it.

Once you have determined the root of your stress, you can create alternative ways of dealing with it. For instance, I am an impatient driver, and driving in today's traffic with the crowded roads and road rage is more difficult than ever. I used to drive as if I were a running back in a football game, constantly looking for openings in the traffic so I could zip through them. I have experienced road rage more times than I would like to admit. I would become so aggravated and angry with the way others drove that it would be impossible for me to carry on a pleasant conversation with my wife while I was driving. She, as you can imagine, was as stressed as I was about my driving.

After experiencing pain in my shoulders and neck as well as elevated blood pressure, I decided to change my perspective. Because it is impossible to change the way others drive, I decided to retire from the game of automobile football. So I slowed down my driving. I leave earlier for my appointments. I am now able to laugh at the frantic driving that I see. With a few deep breaths and good music on the stereo, driving has become a pleasurable new experience for me.

I identified the stressful event—driving. My impatience was the root of my stress. By changing my perspective toward traffic, I now drive with much less stress.

Changing our stressful habits can really aid us in reducing tension in our lives. But we also need to actively practice positive techniques such as progressive relaxation in order to de-stress.

17

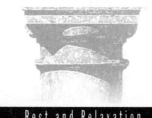

Rest and Relaxation

PROGRESSIVE RELAXATION

Stress management activities should become a part of our everyday lives. They reduce the level of anxiety and emotional distress we may be experiencing and help us release the negative buildup that is destroying our health.

As you get relief from the following techniques, I hope you will incorporate them into your daily life, because they will help you feel good and have much more energy. Consider spending some time—in the mornings before you start your day off or at night after the kids are in bed—doing these stress relievers so you can start your day off right or get a good night's sleep.

BREATHING

WHEN I FIRST started practicing this technique, I did it to help my powerlifting. I didn't realize it was custom-made for channeling my stress and my anxieties. Your reasons for learning to relax are probably not the same as mine, but I encourage you to try this breathing technique. Perhaps it will bring you stress relief, too.

Find a comfortable position on the floor or in a chair and just allow your body to go limp (while sitting upright). Then force yourself to inhale slowly for as long as you can. Hold it for a second, then exhale all the air out of your lungs just as slowly. Aim for one slow inhale and one slow exhale every minute, forcing all the air out of your lungs each time.

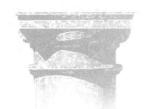

This breathing technique will help reduce your blood pressure heart rate and pulse, plus it will calm the muscles that are tight from tension and stress.

Don't be disappointed if you cannot make one cycle of breathing last sixty seconds. You will most likely have to build up to it, but in the process you will learn how to relax your body at will. As you inhale, picture white arrows (representing oxygen) entering your throat, then your lungs. When you exhale, picture black arrows leaving your body, ridding it of toxins and carbon dioxide. Try this breathing exercise for five minutes at a time.

This breathing technique will help reduce your blood pressure, heart rate and pulse, plus it will calm the muscles that are tight from tension and stress.

You might want to practice this breathing technique when the kids are in bed or when nobody is around to disturb you. After you master this breathing technique, it won't matter where you are because you can do it anywhere, anytime.

This relaxation exercise will be very beneficial to you, particularly if you have speaking engagements, have to perform before a crowd, have an interview for a job or a salary increase or just need to slow things down in the middle of the day. It will put your body and mind in a very calming mood.

MUSCLE TENSING

WHEN I WAS in the military, I was stationed on Okinawa. I remember driving by office buildings and seeing the employees outside doing a

HEALTH **FACT** BOX

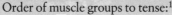

Order of muscle groups to tense:[1]
- Clench your right fist. This relaxes the right hand and forearm.
- Clench your left fist. This relaxes the left hand and forearm.
- Clench both fists.
- Bend both wrists.
- Frown. This relaxes the forehead and scalp.
- Squint your eyes. This relaxes the eye muscles and the face.
- Clench your teeth. This relaxes the jaw.
- Push back against the headrest. This relaxes the neck.
- Shrug your shoulders. This relaxes the shoulders and back.
- Take a deep breath. Hold it, then forcefully exhale. This relaxes the chest.
- Tighten your abdominal (stomach) muscles.
- Tighten your buttocks, thighs and calves all at once. This relaxes the lower extremities.
- Point your toes forward. This relaxes the foot muscles.

series of stretches and calisthenics. Often companies had mid-morning, noon and midafternoon breaks just for this purpose. That was great stress management!

Muscle tensing can bring relaxation to our bodies, too. Called progressive muscle relaxation, this process is simply working with one muscle group at a time by tensing the muscle for eight to ten seconds and then releasing the tension. You will feel the tension leave as you do this. Try to perform these exercises when nobody is around to interrupt the session. You can sit while you do these exercises. If you prefer to lie on the floor, roll up a towel and place it under your neck for support. Each session should last about ten to fourteen minutes.

Prepare for your session by getting comfortable. Take off your shoes and loosen your belt and tie—or remove them. Remove your glasses or contacts if you wear them. Then close your eyes and relax the best you can (the breathing technique can help here) for a minute or two. Then take the following steps:

1. Working with one muscle group at a time, tense each muscle group two times for fifteen seconds each time. Do it in the order listed in the Healthfact box and move at a slow pace.

2. Pause and take deep breaths intermittently.

3. Contract your muscles at approximately 60 to 70 percent of maximum output, or until they are fairly tight.

When you are finished, take a deep breath. Hold, then forcefully exhale. As you exhale say, "Relax." This mental reinforcement improves your concentration and helps you relax even more. Rest for two to three minutes, then get up.

Autogenic Training

When I was competing in powerlifting, I had to do three lifts of maximum weight that were tallied to come up with the total combined poundage. These lifts included the bench press, the squat and the dead lift, and the more weight I could lift, the better.

After doing all the physical strength programs for powerlifting, as well as learning lifting techniques and style, I still needed an edge for the mental side of the sport. I learned about having a positive mental attitude, but I had to go beyond positive thinking. That's when I learned about autogenic training, or mental imagery.

In my case, the goal was to envision the perfect squatting technique. Trust me, when you are standing with a 750-pound barbell draped over your shoulders that is compressing your vertebrae and discs with tens of thousands of pounds per square inch, good technique goes a long way. Autogenic training helped me with the competitions, and it relaxed me as well.

Autogenic training is simply using mental exercises to trigger the relaxation response. It does not use outside stimuli, but is solely a mental exercise. This training produces sensations of warmth and heaviness, which are calming and soothing. It has been successful in treating people who have high blood pressure, migraine headaches, asthma and sleep disturbances.

Get in any position you want as long as you are comfortable. Now, focus on mental pictures of a place or of scenery you find to be very tranquil or very lovely. Perhaps you remember a vista you saw once while on vacation, or maybe you recall a beautiful scene from a book or a painting. For you, the perfect scene may be a still lake surrounded by huge snow-capped mountains, or perhaps a view from an airplane of the billowy white clouds below you. Maybe it's lying on the white sand beach of a tropical island or floating in the warm ocean. For me, it's that hammock in Jamaica!

If you are lying on a mattress, imagine that you are sinking deep into it. Hold your image as the focus point of your thoughts for as long as you can. This encourages deeper relaxation.

Do this as often as you need to. As you practice this technique, you will find it easier and easier to move into a relaxing state of mind quickly. Then it will be natural to fall into a good sleep, which is what we want to talk about next.

18

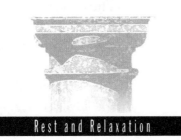

A Good Night's Rest

I cherish my sleep. How about you?

The average person spends about one-third of his or her life asleep. That might sound like a waste of a lot of good hours! You could be doing something else more productive—golfing, training or making a buck, right? No, sleep is actually productive time because your body regenerates itself through sleep.

Rebuilding Your Health Through Sleep

Two basic types of people exist today. One type spends their health in the attempt to gain wealth. These people eventually must spend all their wealth to regain their health. The other type is more balanced. They spend energy and time building a secure future, while at the same time trying to maintain a healthy lifestyle.

Yet both lifestyles, when pushed to the limit, can stress the body and shortchange its health. Our bodies are capable of handling just so much physical work and mental and emotional strain. Then they need to recharge with a good night's sleep.

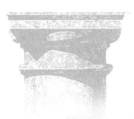

Those precious hours under the covers are exactly what our bodies need for optimum efficiency.

Your nighttime sleeping patterns can be disrupted by living your life in the Overload Zone for too long. Too much stress, constant anxiety and poor dietary habits can interfere with a good night's sleep. Actually, even doing good things such as physical exercise or training can interfere with your deep-sleep patterns. The more intense your workouts, the more adjustments your body has to make.

Sleep is actually productive time because your body regenerates itself through sleep.

Research shows that sleeping every night is one of the most important things we can do for our health. While we are sleeping, not doing much in the way of activities, our bodies are hard at work repairing and rebuilding. During sleep, at a specific time, the body produces and releases hormones and neurotransmitters to repair and rebuild itself. Generally, this time is when the individual reaches rapid-eye movement (REM) sleep. But if REM is not reached, then these metabolic processes are interrupted, and a breakdown in health begins.

As we already learned, building lean muscle weight is ideal for many reasons. But you will find it interesting that it is not during your workouts that your muscles grow. They actually grow while you sleep. The process of growth and repair of muscles is regulated by a number of neurotransmitters and hormones. The orchestra leader in charge of this biochemical band is melatonin.

Melatonin

Melatonin, a hormone that is released by a tiny pea-sized gland in our brains called the pineal gland, is responsible for setting our internal clocks. The sleep-wake cycle is directly linked to the precise timing of the release of this hormone.

As our bodies age, they produce less melatonin, which causes them to no longer reach the deep state of sleep they did when they were younger. And as we learned, reaching that deep sleep state is necessary for the body to rebuild and repair itself.

The amount of deep sleep we get, along with the amount of melatonin that is released, affects the release of other biochemicals, such as HGH (human growth hormone), DHEA, cortisol and the steroid hormones. These hormones stimulate immune function, muscle growth, tissue repair and a myriad of other essential processes.[1]

Our Creator saw fit to design and program His human creation to have their sleep-wake cycle coincide with day and night. Darkness is directly responsible for the release of melatonin, which peaks around 2:00 A.M. and returns to the baseline at approximately 8:00 A.M. The problem is, we don't always listen to our bodies, so sometimes we don't get the sleep we need.

Have you ever pulled an all-nighter? Staying up all night creates a significant challenge to the immune system. Studies have shown that getting inadequate sleep can interfere with the normal release of HGH—and less HGH speeds up the aging process.

Over time, if you are not getting that full night's sleep for whatever reason, your body will start suppressing your melatonin secretions. This, in turn, will play havoc with your body's hormonal balance. When this pattern of being up all night becomes the rule instead of the exception, this sleep debt will eventually catch up with you.

During the daytime, your reaction time will be slower, your brain will feel fogged out, and you won't make good decisions. If you are not getting enough sleep, you will be sleepy and fatigued during the day. Most people think that drinking several cups of coffee does the

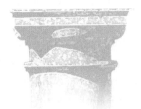

Missing sleep night after night will weaken your immune system. Before you realize it, you will have caught every bug that is flying around the office.

trick. Sorry, that won't help. Your body is fatigued because you missed the sleep.

With this in mind, if you plan to buy a car anytime in the near future, remember not to buy one that was built on a Monday! All the weekend warriors and party animals are on the assembly line Monday morning, probably sleepy and fatigued from their weekends.

Missing sleep night after night will weaken your immune system. Before you realize it, you will have caught every bug that is flying around the office. Eventually this sleep debt may increase the chances of heart disease and osteoporosis because of the hormonal imbalance that results.

You must get enough deep rest every night for good health.

Developing Good Sleeping Habits

It's important to do whatever it takes to get a good night's rest. For years Lori and I have worked out of our home. Those of you familiar with a home-based business know that the phone can ring at any time. So, in order to protect our sleep, I decided to unplug the phone in our bedroom at night. That way the recorder takes a message, and we get a good night's sleep.

The beginning of good sleeping habits is going to bed at the same time each night and waking up at the same time each morning. Perhaps you have heard people say they are morning people or night people. What does a married couple do when one spouse is a night person and the other is a morning person?

Lori and I are opposites like that. She finds it difficult to go to bed before midnight, and I could go to bed at 10:00 P.M. She loves to sleep in, and I couldn't sleep in if my life depended on it. She needs something to stop her mind from thinking so she can fall asleep. I am asleep on the way down to the pillow. She will count to herself, read or watch TV while I'm already in dreamland.

So, how can two people like us hit the hay at the same time?

A couple years ago I decided to take melatonin at night before I went to bed. I didn't need it to fall asleep, even though it did seem to relax me. I started taking it because, as we learned, our bodies produce less melatonin as we age, whether we exercise and eat healthy foods or not. So as a preventative measure, I thought it was a wise idea to add melatonin to my daily dietary supplement regime.

Shortly after I started taking it, I noticed the benefits it brought. So I suggested that Lori start taking it. Well, it worked. Now, one hour before she plans to go to bed, she takes melatonin. Then at bedtime, she finds herself ready for sleep. It works great!

You might want to consider adding this dietary supplementation to your new healthy lifestyle. Of course, the dosages are different for different people, so I suggest that you talk with a nutritional pro for advice. However, remember that melatonin is a powerful neurohormone that should not be used in a haphazard manner.[2]

Insomnia and Chemical Complications

ONE OF THE most aggravating frustrations that people can experience is insomnia—not being able to fall asleep, no matter how tired they are. Mental exercises, such as counting sheep or thinking in circles, only frustrate the problem. No wonder there are so many sleep medications prescribed for the non-sleeper.

Studies in sleep labs have shown that insomniacs need more time to enter the first stage of sleep than others do.[3] Additionally, often the REM state and the dream state of insomniacs are disrupted because of the individuals' erratic sleeping patterns.

They toss and turn, awakening frequently, and often arise feeling as though they had no rest.

Many insomniacs take sleeping pills, but sleeping medications can interfere with REM sleep, alter sleep patterns and induce chemical dependency. Consequently, people who take these chemicals regularly may never be fully rested. Plus, after a period of time, the body builds immunity to the medications and requires more, thus creating problems of addiction.

Other people may have some alcohol to calm them down at the end of a busy day. But drinking alcohol before bedtime actually prevents a person from entering into REM sleep and can cause nighttime hypoglycemia, which is a very common cause for awakening at night.[4]

Perhaps you've heard a person who drank too much the night before say, "I slept like a log last night." Not a chance! REM sleep was never reached, so that person did not wake up the next morning fully rested. That's often obvious to everyone but the person himself!

Another reason insomniacs find it hard to sleep is that they think they need more sleep than they actually require. Deep REM sleep is what is required for rest and recovery, not necessarily the old standard of eight to ten hours of any kind of sleep. In reality, what insomniacs need is better nutrition. The better the nutrition through compatible food selections and dietary supplements, the less sleep the body needs.

You might want to skip late-night eating, which causes the digestive system to kick into overtime. That will ruin your chances of a sound sleep. It is better to lean toward being slightly hungry on the way to bed than cleaning food from your teeth.

If you find it difficult to sleep at night, try avoiding any caffeine late in the day. Remember that caffeine comes in teas, sodas and chocolate as well as coffee.

A Good Night's Rest

Natural Sleep Aids

Tests have shown that certain nutrients can induce and help maintain sleep. Nature has fascinating ways of helping our bodies repair, rebuild, relax and rejuvenate without the use of medication or drugs. When used in their proper amounts, the following nutrients can be helpful for sleep.

Calcium plays an important role to calm nervousness and restlessness, thereby helping us sleep. Children who are hyperactive have been known to experience a calming effect from calcium supplementation. The best way to take calcium is with magnesium. Calcium and magnesium work most effectively in a dosage of two parts calcium to one part magnesium.

Magnesium plays a huge role in normalizing the activity of the nerves. It stores itself in the skeletal muscles and promotes the necessary stimuli for muscular control and relaxation. Magnesium also protects muscles from cramping.

Hops is regarded as a powerful, stimulating and relaxing nerve tonic. It is good for cardiovascular disorders, yet it produces soothing rest for anxiety, hyperactivity, insomnia, nervousness, restlessness and stress. Hops relaxes the liver and gall ducts, and even serves as a mild laxative. Some people find that placing it inside a pillowcase aids sleep.[5]

Chamomile is a natural sedative. It is a traditional remedy for stress, anxiety, indigestion and insomnia.

Alfalfa contains powerful trace minerals. It also contains vitamin A and enzymes that assist the body in digestion. It helps sleep indirectly by calming the digestive tract, also providing some relief from peptic ulcers, kidney and bladder problems as well as pain relief from arthritis.

Inositol is a member of the B family and has been proven to help patients sleep, according to Dr. Robert C. Atkins, M.D.[6]

Pantothenic acid is a member of the B vitamin family and works well with inositol for relaxation.

L-tryptophan is not a vitamin but an amino acid (one of nature's building blocks from which protein is made). Your body does not manufacture it, so you need to supplement it with your diet. Have you ever felt sleepy after eating turkey? Well, that's because turkey is a good source of tryptophan.

Niacinamide is another member of the B vitamin family and enhances the effects of tryptophan.

HEALTH **FACT** BOX

NATURAL SLEEP AIDS

- Calcium
- Magnesium
- Hops
- Chamomile
- Alfalfa
- Inositol
- Pantothenic acid
- L-tryptophan
- Niacinamide

When you experiment with natural dietary supplements as alternatives to pharmaceutical sleep inducers, you will find they work opposite from the drugs. Barbiturates prescribed for sleeping purposes usually start with lower dosages and must be increased as the body becomes addicted to the drugs.

But with dietary supplements, you might need to take heavier amounts at first in order to help get your body healthy and functioning properly. Then, after your body is healed and has improved bodily performance and function, the dosages often can be reduced to a minimum. In many cases, they won't be needed at all.

Anxiety is somewhat related to insomnia. The nutrients that are helpful for one are also helpful for the other.

Sleep It Up!

THE IMPORTANCE OF getting regular sleep cannot be stressed enough. Sleep deprivation leads to hormonal imbalance, which in turn disrupts the body's ability to repair itself and rebuild muscle tissue. Without sleep, the body cannot meet its other hormonal needs. Plus, the aging process is speeded up—and who wants that?

On the other hand, reestablishing your sleep-wake cycle will enhance your health and your body's ability to recover from stress and anxiety. Plus, you will have the ability to perform at your optimum.

So sleep it up!

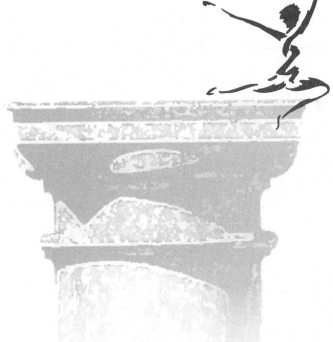

Anti-Aging Strategies

7

His days will be a hundred and

twenty years.

—Genesis 6:3

PILLAR SEVEN

19

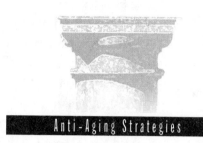

Anti-Aging Strategies

AGING AND DETERIORATION

According to Ashley Montagu, "The goal is to die young—as late as possible."

If you're reading this book, there's a good chance you are a baby boomer—an American born between 1946 and 1964. Baby boomers equaled one-third of our country's entire population during those years.

Ken Dychtwalk, Ph.D., stated "As teenagers, boomers bought 43 percent of records sold, 53 percent of movie tickets and 55 percent of sodas. Four years later, the colleges were overwhelmed by the number of people enrolling. Ten years later, the housing market was stunned by the number of people buying first homes. The first of the boomers are now turning fifty. *Every eight seconds one of them is receiving an invitation from the American Association of Retired Persons.*"[1]

The majority of baby boomers will turn sixty-five between the years 2010 and 2030. As this generation enters old age, you can bank on the fact that they are not going to just roll over and die, but will fight every inch of the way to retain that youthfulness they remember so well.

Seven Pillars of Health

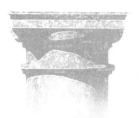

This aging generation, along with the growing numbers in the senior marketplace, is not accepting the over-the-hill mentality. Instead, they are changing the meaning of fitness.

How will baby boomers deal with aging? Author Jeff Ostroff exposes the heartbeat of the boomer generation. "Having built their identity as America's youth generation, the boomers will not enter the second 50 years of life with a whimper. Instead, they'll do everything they can to delay or counteract the effects of aging."[2]

This aging generation, along with the growing numbers in the senior marketplace, is not accepting the over-the-hill mentality. Instead, they are changing the meaning of fitness. The baby boom market is predicted to have tremendous growth over the next decades, especially in the healthcare and fitness service areas. That's because fighting the aging process has become the number one target for this huge section of our population. Those who once possessed the curvaceous figures and Adonis-like bodies will not submit to the aging process without a fight. They will not give in to the mentality that life is over after forty.

With the greater percentage of boomers turning fifty, older adults are now the fastest-growing segment in the U.S. population today.[3] According to the United Nations Population Division, this age wave is expected to continue well into the middle of this century.[4]

In 1900, there were about 75.9 million Americans. At the end of 1999, there are 75.9 million Americans *over the age of fifty.*[5]

I have always envisioned being around in the mid-twenty-first century. I think it would be extraordinary to tell stories to the young fifty-year-old fitness enthusiasts at the gym then. Watching their expressions will be priceless when I tell them about living back in the medieval days, when television came only in black and white. But I want to be in good health when I talk to them. Dr. Robert Butter, CEO of the International Longevity Center, states, "While ideas about aging are improving, Americans still need to do a better job of preparing for old age."[6]

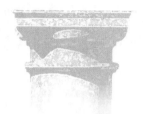

Today, approximately 80 percent of older Americans reportedly suffer from some form of chronic back pain.[7] Millions of others experience the day-to-day nagging pain of arthritis

When your health is upside down, everything you have going on in your life comes to a screeching halt!

in the knees, hips and hands. Many have orthopedic conditions as well as other ailments.

Yet living longer and healthier is the forecast for the boomers. Most are expecting to go through their later years more youthfully than the previous generation did because they will work harder at it. I'm not suggesting that we will not experience pain or discomfort in our aging years, but to be crippled because of lack of effort or laziness is our own fault. I have always said that I would rather check out of life at ninety miles per hour than be forced to use a walker for the last twenty years due to neglecting and abusing my body.

I don't presume my tomorrows are guaranteed. So I am of the belief that if people make regular exercise, eating foods compatible to their blood type and dietary supplements a constant part of their lives, they will live longer. There's an article in the paper almost daily giving evidence that that we can increase our life spans by doing these things.

As we age, we all should have the desire to create a greater quality of life for ourselves and our loved ones. When your health is upside down, everything you have going on in your life comes to a screeching halt!

HEALTH **FACT** BOX

The aging process actually begins when a person is in his or her twenties and thirties. Most people soar through their next ten to twenty years either ignoring or being unaware of the fact that their bodies are aging. Then they reach their forties, when many of the anti-aging hormones drop off significantly. Finally, when people reach their fifties and sixties, they indeed start feeling and seeing the effects of natural aging.

Is Deterioration Inevitable?

PAIN IN THE joints—the knees, ankles, hips, shoulders, elbows and spine—is a malady associated with aging. The joints are connected and attached with soft tissue, referred to as ligaments, and tendons, which connect the bone to muscle. Unfortunately, our joints can undergo some severe damage and destruction from falls, accidents, sports-related injuries—or just from the aging process itself.

Years ago during a powerlifting training session, I was attempting to lift 700 pounds. Somehow, my right foot slipped about two inches, and I felt immediate pain in my right knee. I went to an orthopedic physician for advice because I had an important competition coming up. He told me that he could shoot the knee with cortisone, but he would do it only once because of the potential damage it could cause to the knee. My response to him was that I was more interested in walking for the rest of my life than squatting one time with 700 pounds on my shoulders! Today, two decades later, my knee causes me pain from time to time. But I can now say that my foolhardy days of powerlifting have been conquered by my brilliant mind!

With time and overuse, the cartilage in a joint starts to degenerate, and the joint can find itself rubbing bone against bone instead of being protected by the soft cartilage. Consequently, the joints can become painful and inflamed from cartilage degeneration as well as osteoporosis and arthritis.

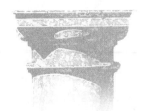

The sad reality is that as people age, they become less physically active. They find themselves sitting more, driving instead of walking, taking the escalator instead of the stairs and doing less than they did when they were younger. This lack

Lack of activity actually contributes to the joint problem, lessening the chance of having healthy joints and making old age painful.

of activity actually contributes to the joint problem, lessening the chance of having healthy joints and making old age painful.

On the other hand, sometimes pain causes the lack of activity. As the human body ages, the joints naturally begin to wear down. Then pain sets in, which causes lifestyle limitations and sometimes disabilities. Because the pain is so great, the individual ceases doing much in the way of activities and consequently, arthritic-like inflammation sets in, which immobilizes and cripples.

That seems to paint a dim picture of aging. The good news is, we can take some preventative and protective measures to strengthen those joints and keep them stable, strong and pain free.

Today, continued research and discoveries point to the idea that the aging process can be prevented and in some cases reversed. Cells can be revitalized and we can gain back some of our youth. But is longevity itself our goal? I believe our goal should be to live as long as

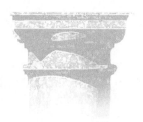

I believe our goal should be to live as long as God gives us breath in as healthy and youthful condition as possible.

God gives us breath *in as healthy and youthful condition as possible.*

It has become common for aging people to suffer from heart attacks, high blood pressure, strokes, cancer, arthritis, Alzheimer's and degenerative diseases. These conditions account for approximately 90 percent of the natural aging process.[8] So it is difficult to imagine that these illnesses might actually be symptoms of something greater taking place.

If we are willing to change our thinking, to quit accepting as gospel the idea that because we are aging we automatically should be suffering, then we have a good chance of living longer with a greater quality of life. It is now thought possible for a person to live to be one hundred or more and still be healthy and full of vitality.

Knowledge is the key to success, and application of it is the power.

What does the baby-boomer generation want as they enter the new millennium? They want to feel good and maintain their youthful appearance, and they are prepared to fight the aging process every step of the way. What they are looking for is quality of life!

The war is on and the battle trumpet has sounded. Let's join the huge segment of today's population who is fighting the aging process.

Chronological Age

When are people considered older adults? Physically, studies show that once people enter their sixth decade, they start losing muscular strength, size and function.[9] The U.S. Census Bureau defines seniors

Aging and Deterioration

as persons sixty-five and older, while many businesses offer discounts for people age fifty-five and older. The American Association of Retired Persons considers anyone fifty years old a senior citizen. In fact, when I turned fifty, I received a gold award checking account from my bank. I guess we have to take 'em where we can get 'em, eh?

America's senior population is getting older all the time. The sixty-five- to seventy-four-age group is eight times larger today than it was in 1900, while the seventy-five- to eighty-four-age group is sixteen times larger. The over-eighty-five-age group is thirty-one times larger.[10] The female population is outgrowing the male population. For example, the average ratio is 143 senior women to every 100 senior men. As age increases, the ratios widen. While there are 119 women to every 100 men at ages sixty-five to sixty-nine, the number increases to 248 to 100 over age eighty-five.[11]

Chronological age is valuable to consider. But evaluating the aging process solely by chronological age has its limitations. That's why we have to look at functional age.

FUNCTIONAL AGE

HAVE YOU EVER seen a sixty-five-year-old man or woman running in a marathon? It's more and more common these days. Then there's the sixty-five-year-old you often help to put his groceries in the car because it's a struggle for him. Both of these people are age sixty-five, yet their functional ages are vastly different.

There is nothing we can do to change our chronological age. Our history on this earth comprises exactly the number of years from the year we were born until today. But as we have observed, chronological age is not an accurate monitoring device to determine a person's true physical condition. The truer measurement of age is what gerontologists call "functional age."

Functional age is determined by looking at the aging-related or

191

disease-related changes that take place in the body and measuring their effects on daily tasks. Heredity, gender, physical injuries, lifestyle and chronic diseases all affect a person's functional age.

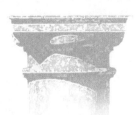

Chronological age is not an accurate monitoring device to determine a person's true physical condition. The truer measurement of age is what gerontologists call "functional age."

An active seventy-year-old who is aging gracefully can have the functional age of a sixty-year-old. On the other hand, a seventy-year-old person who has been hampered with illness or multiple medical problems may have the functional age of an eighty-year-old.

Functional age is also affected by the attitude of the aging adults. People who hit the age of forty are told they are over the hill. We have to be careful not to accept this idea, even subconsciously, because it can cause our state of mind to do just that: go downhill. We can now stay youthful and live a life free of diseases well into our later years, so our chronological age has loosened its once strong hold on us.

It has been my experience that as people reach midlife and start taking care of their bodies and their health, they not only begin functioning physically as they did when they were younger, but they also develop the more youthful and vibrant mental attitude that goes along with it.

I have always said that if people would make regular exercise, sensible eating and dietary supplements part of their everyday lives, they would have to think hard when asked how old they are. Reports have suggested that men and women who are athletically and nutritionally fit can actually function as many as ten to twenty years younger than their chronological age.

Aging and Deterioration

Let me give you an example.

My wife, Lori, and I went out for dinner one evening with an older couple who were friends of Lori's. During dinner the husband shared with me how he loves to exercise. Three days a week he drives to the YMCA and does thirty minutes of swimming, forty-five minutes of water aerobics and then attends a forty-five-minute aerobic class in the gym. He said he has never felt better in life. His mind is sharp, he takes his supplements daily, and he has lots of energy. He is thrilled that he started exercising fifteen years ago.

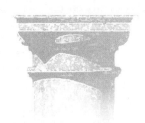

I have always said that if people would make regular exercise, sensible eating and dietary supplements part of their everyday lives, they would have to think hard when asked how old they are.

When he said that, I did some quick mental calculations. I knew he was ninety years young. That meant this little Hercules sitting across from me had started all that exercising fifteen years ago when he was seventy-five! His functional age was certainly quite a bit lower than his chronological age.

That's the goal—getting our functional age as low as possible. So as we age, keep in mind that those who exercise have a lower functional age than those who do not. Plus, after the age of twenty-five, the sedentary person loses approximately one-half pound of muscle per year. By the age of seventy, about 40 percent of muscle mass is lost if muscle activation or stimulation is not applied.[12]

Senior Functional Classifications

To determine age by functional capacity, a functional classification has been developed.[13]

Seven Pillars of Health

Physically elite. This group represents a very small percentage of seniors. They train on a daily basis and compete in sports such as the Senior Olympics or triathlons. Or they participate regularly in vigorous activities or group fitness classes. These seniors can participate in high-risk activities like weightlifting and usually perform at the highest level.

Physically fit. This is a larger group than the elite group, but it is still a small percentage of the population. These seniors typically participate in exercise sessions at least two times per week. They venture out and do some rollerblading or play tennis. They are capable of participating in endurance sports like powerwalking, and they are at low risk for falling into the "physically frail" category.

Physically independent. This group of seniors shows signs of loss in balance, coordination, strength and flexibility. They are the largest group of seniors and range from fairly active to somewhat functionally independent. They may engage in crafts or gardening and perhaps take light walks. They participate in low-level activities such as playing golf. They don't show any debilitating symptoms, but an injury or illness could affect their mobility and physical function. They are apt to fall into the "physically frail" category.

Physically frail. These seniors perform daily activities that are not very demanding, such as shopping and cleaning. They are capable of light activities, but usually sit around and watch television. In many cases, they just stay at home.

Physically dependent. This group represents a small percentage of seniors who are often in wheelchairs and need home care. Basically, they spend much of their money on healthcare.

Totally disabled. This small group of seniors cannot stand or walk. They must rely on complete assistance from a professional healthcare staff.

Reading these categories is sobering, isn't it? So let's find out how we can fight the aging process.

20

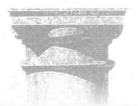

BEATING THE AGING PROCESS WITH EXERCISE

T he closest thing to the anti-aging pill is exercise," says Dr. Alex Leif from Harvard Medical School.[1]

Regular physical activity can help the body maintain, repair and improve itself. Older people, even those who are disabled or ill, can and should take part in some form of exercise program. Exercise strengthens the heart and lungs, lowers blood pressure and protects against the onset of adult diabetes. It builds, tones and strengthens muscles and keeps the joints and tendons more flexible. Physical activity gives people more energy, lessens tension and anxiety and also improves sleep. All in all, exercise contributes to longevity.

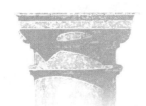

Exercise can strengthen bones, thereby slowing down the process of osteoporosis.

Research shows that exercise is an important key component for preventing and treating heart disease, osteoporosis, frailty, diabetes, obesity and depression. Exercise can be an effective weapon in the fight against these diseases.

HEALTH **FACT** BOX

- **Fighting osteoporosis.** Exercise can strengthen bones, thereby slowing down the process of osteoporosis. Exercising thirty to sixty minutes three times weekly can help fight osteoporosis.
- **Fighting coronary heart disease.** A combination of strength training and aerobic training will increase the strength and efficiency of the heart muscles. A strong heart eases the workload. If the heart doesn't have to work as hard, it will probably last longer.
- **Fighting noninsulin-dependent diabetes.** The body's ability to use glucose slows down with age. Exercise is a natural preventative that may increase insulin sensitivity, which helps keep blood glucose levels under control for the long haul.
- **Fighting obesity.** Body weight is best controlled with the combination of proper diet and regular exercise. An individual who is obese and physically inactive must be selective in choosing an exercise program. Even walking can be difficult, so a gradual but consistent approach should be applied.
- **Fighting frailty.** Frailty in older people can be reversed with regular exercise. People in their mideighties to midnineties who exercise and strengthen their muscles experience more stability and endurance.
- **Fighting poor mental health.** Exercise has been shown to improve one's self image and to provide a way to vent built-up anxieties, tensions, depression and fears.

Beating the Aging Process With Exercise

Not Pain, but Gain

This MATURING GENERATION of boomers is becoming a fitness-conscious people, but they are not interested in the no-pain, no-gain mentality. They are striving for a low-impact to no-impact type of exercising. The boomer is looking for a workout that will save the joints and at the same time produce high energy. The focus is on a better quality of life.

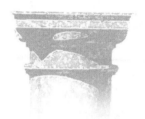

Even though I am a former national competitive powerlifter and bodybuilder, I no longer care to compete with the "big boys" at the gym. I am pleased to measure up to my own standards for an energetic and disease-free life that allows me to enjoy life and accommodate my

The boomer is looking for a workout that will save the joints and at the same time produce high energy. The focus is on a better quality of life.

family—including my grandchildren. It is important to me that "Papa Joe" be a picture of vitality and health rather than some withered-away fixture that my grandkids see every Sunday afternoon sunken into the easy chair.

So, fitness for the boomer is growing more diverse. As the search for social fulfillment in the later years grows, so do the fitness options. These options include:

Over-fifty sports leagues and group activities, such as tennis, golfing, bowling, water aerobics, walking and bicycling should become an continuing part of the aging boomer's life.

Cardiovascular workouts are absolutely necessary for burning the unwanted layers of fat and keeping the ticker healthy. It is estimated that nearly five million people a year are diagnosed with coronary heart disease.[2] The prevention of this disease and the maintenance of a healthy body weight requires incorporating a form of regular cardiovascular exercise either daily or every other day. My suggestion—and the Surgeon General's suggestion—is thirty minutes a day of exercise.

Exercises that target balance and coordination, motor flexibility and improvement in posture are more important after age fifty. Water workouts are very effective for obtaining these improvements.

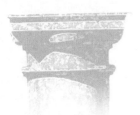

Strength training is now more recognized than ever for its positive impact on retaining strong, healthy muscles. It's amazing that as people age, some are fortunate enough to dodge the heart attack bullet, only to die from a fall. Physicians and Sports

Since the nineties there has been a shift in emphasis from cardiovascular training to strength training.

Medicine reports that 40 percent of adults over the age of sixty-five fall at least once a year.[3] Subsequently, strength training is becoming a part of the boomers' workouts.

Strength training, also called resistance training, is no longer limited just to the bodybuilder. In fact, everyone can benefit from strength training. The American College of Sports Medicine places more emphasis on strength training than any other type, incorporating it in aerobic training for a well-rounded training program.

Since the nineties there has been a shift in emphasis from cardiovascular training to strength training. Traditionally, medical experts have focused much of their attention on cardiovascular training for improved health and reduction in heart disease. But these older guidelines ignored the musculoskeletal system.

Problems associated with the musculoskeletal system create a new concern for aging adults who want to keep their functional independence. For instance, as people age, their bodies becomes more fragile because activity levels decrease. This is compounded by a loss in bone and muscle mass. If we do not use our bodies, we will lose them! For many people, the problem isn't aging—it's disuse. Barry Franklin, Ph.D., president of the American College of Sports Medicine, states, "People who don't exercise regularly suffer a 1 percent loss in aerobic fitness every year starting at age twenty. But that loss can be restored years later through three months of steady walking, jogging or biking."[4]

Many health professionals today are agreeing that strength training might actually be preferred over aerobic training and other activities as the most effective means of countering the aging process.

Today the YMCA workout rooms and even some of the gyms are graced with people in their seventies, eighties and nineties. *Modern Maturity* reports, "Whether chasing gold medals or running around the neighborhood, 50-plus America is on the move. More and more people are toning up, slimming down, and attaining a fitness level belying their years."[5]

Many health professionals today are agreeing that strength training might actually be preferred over aerobic training and other activities as the most effective means of countering the aging process.

As we live longer and face the challenges of aging, I believe strength training is going to be the key that will help seniors improve their health, functional capacities, quality of life and independent lifestyle.

Let me give you an example of the effect strength training is having on older adults.

Seven Pillars of Health

JACK AND JUNE

I HAVE BEEN training a husband and wife for several years. Jack is sixty-seven years old and a blood type O, and June is sixty-six years old and a blood type AB. It's been a pleasure to see this couple grind it out every other day each week for months and months. Their tenacity and persistent attitude about keeping physical fitness a consistent component of their lifestyle is a true asset and a joy to witness.

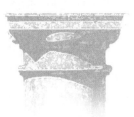

Not only has her body taken on a healthier and more youthful look, but her energy level is that of women thirty years younger. She is a true example of what functional age is all about.

At first June was the one who wanted to get in shape. Then Jack decided to get with the program. June is very active with plenty of energy to burn. She operates her own interior design business out of her home and is constantly on the go, giving estimates, designing furniture and overseeing installations. Many days she works until 6 or 7 P.M.

In order to make time to exercise before her day begins, June meets with me at 7:15 A.M. three days a week. She starts out her program by spending anywhere from fifteen to twenty-five minutes on her treadmill. After she has a good sweat going, we begin.

She trains for approximately forty-five minutes, combining a cardiovascular workout with circuit weight training. At first, we selected weights that were at the beginners' level. But as she has progressed over the years, she has become quite a strong lifter.

Not only has her body taken on a healthier and more youthful look, but her energy level is that of women thirty years younger. She is a true example of what functional age is all about.

200

Beating the Aging Process With Exercise

Jack is completely different from his wife. He is a big man and enjoys building muscle and getting strong. At 8:00 A.M., three days a week, he likes to grind out those heavy-weighted sets of curls, shoulder presses and dumbbell chest presses. When he and I first began his fitness journey, he was using a fifteen-pound dumbbell for bicep curls and chest presses. Today he can handle those big twenty-five-pound and thirty-pound dumb-bells for curling with ease. In fact, he had to purchase heavier dumbbells because of his progressive strength and muscle gains! He likes to throw around those forty-pound dumbbells on the chest press exercises. With a big grin on his face, he says the only problem he has had from all the strength training is that he can't fit into his suits anymore.

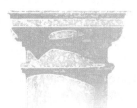

With a big grin on his face, he says the only problem he has had from all the strength training is that he can't fit into his suits anymore.

I find it to be true that older adults who are exercising regularly and doing strength training as a major part of their routine are surpassing all their peers in their sports and recreational activities. Plus, what makes my day about Jack and June is that their physical activity and fitness level carries over to their mental attitude. They have a youthful and joyous attitude toward life.

Strength training provides so many benefits that it should be a part of your Anti-Aging Strategies Pillar if you desire a better quality of life through your later years—and who doesn't?

THE BENEFITS OF STRENGTH TRAINING

THE BENEFITS OF strength training seem to keep increasing. Here are a few:

Metabolism increases and body composition changes. When

strength training, the body burns calories more efficiently. As people develop additional muscle mass, their basal metabolic rate (BMR), or the body's ability to burn more calories at rest, increases. This helps maintain a healthy weight. Plus, with strength training, people have more muscle mass and less fat. Strength training overcomes sarcopenia, or muscle loss.

Functional ability grows. Strength training makes everyday tasks easier and helps people keep their independence.

Arthritic-like pain and disability lessens. Strength training strengthens joints and increases joint lubrication and stability.

Bones become stronger. Strength training fights osteoporosis by increasing bone mineral density. The increased strength of bones, muscles and connective tissue causes a decrease in the risk of injury.

The mind becomes healthier. Strength training improves mental alertness and self-worth, which fights depression—a condition that has become more and more common among our seniors.

Insulin sensitivity improves. Strength training improves insulin sensitivity and glucose regulation, which stabilizes blood sugar. This contributes to a steady energy level.

A greater quality of life and extended functional independence is experienced. As a general rule, people who maintain their physical strength are able to perform everyday activities and tasks much easier and well past their retirement days.

Helping the Joints

If you are the typical mature adult or aging boomer, you are probably experiencing joint pain. The two worst things you can do for your joints is believing that medication will fix them and living a sedentary life. I have counseled many older clients who end up having stomach disorders from taking anti-inflammatory medication for their arthritic pain. The problem then becomes twofold: They have stomach problems in addition to joint pain.

HEALTH **FACT** BOX

THE BENEFITS OF STRENGTH TRAINING

- Metabolism increases and body composition changes.
- Functional ability grows.
- Arthritic-like pain and disability lessens.
- Bones become stronger.
- The mind becomes healthier.
- Insulin sensitivity improves.
- A greater quality of life and extended functional independence is experienced.

The catch is, they are in so much pain that they cannot do anything, so they are forced to live a sedentary life. Then their condition will not improve because they remain inactive, and their lives become nothing more than a day-to-day battle of pain and anguish.

When people are inactive, their muscles atrophy, or weaken in size and strength. Consequently, all the strain and pressure is directly on the joint. So strengthening the muscles and soft tissue that support the joint is part of the plan to rebuild and strengthen the joints.

Here are some preventative and protective measures to take:

Exercise. Have I said enough about exercise yet? Exercise will strengthen the muscles, ligaments and tendons, which directly strengthen the joints and ease the pain.

Exercise the major muscle groups—legs, back, chest, shoulders, abs and arms. Exercise each muscle group two to three times per week. Perform eight to ten repetitions for three sets per exercise.

203

You can utilize free weights or weight machines, as well as flexible stretch cords or bands.

Crunches, not sit-ups, are excellent exercises for strengthening the stomach muscles and do not require any particular piece of equipment. As you strengthen the abdominal muscles, you indirectly make your lower back healthier, stronger and pain free. A strong abdominal wall also stabilizes the movements of your upper torso or trunk.

Stretching. Stretching is necessary for developing and increasing range of motion (ROM) around the joint. Joints become stiff, sore and short-ranged when they are not active and not stretched. Increasing the ROM will increase blood circulation, keep the joint lubricated, enhance everyday tasks, help prevent muscle injuries and make enjoying life with exciting activities more likely.

Static stretching is recommended because it is a gentle form of stretching. Stretch the legs, arms or back to the point where the muscles feel comfortably tight. Hold that position for least fifteen seconds, then return to a relaxed position. Repeat this stretching technique two to three times.

Be sure to breathe freely. Do not hold your breath. The idea is to relax your body so the muscles will elongate and open the range of motion of the joint. Stretching can be done daily, especially before and after exercising.

Starting an Anti-Aging Exercise Program

If you are under thirty-five and in good health, you probably don't need to see a doctor before beginning your exercise program. But if you are over thirty-five and have been inactive for several years, you should consult your physician first. At any age, if you have or have had high blood pressure, dizzy spells, arthritis, heart trouble, ligament or tendon problems or a family history of heart attacks, then you should consult your doctor before beginning your program.

If you are planning to embark on a strength training program but are not quite sure where to begin, let me give you a few suggestions:

Try interviewing some personal trainers at your local YMCA or health clubs. Get references from people you trust. Ask them to do an evaluation of your exercise history, medical history, goals and likes and dislikes pertaining to exercise. Then discuss which activities or exercises will best suit your interests. The more you enjoy the exercises you do, the greater the likelihood of success.

If you do not contact a trainer or exercise consultant, then try the following. Start out by performing two sets of eight to twelve repetitions for basic strength building of the major muscle groups—thighs, back, chest, shoulders, arms and abdominals. The amount of weight or resistance you select should be enough to feel challenging by the end of each set. When you perform each exercise, never hold your breath, but simply breathe as freely as you can.

Full range of motion throughout each exercise will provide a complete stimulus per muscle trained. If the last set of an exercise is completed with ease, that's your indication to move up in the weight or resistance. Usually a 5 to 10 percent increase will suffice.

Allow your level of fitness to dictate how much to do under all circumstances. If you try to do too much at the beginning, you will simply slow down your progress.

Have fun with it. Mix it up. Do some weights one week, then some machines another. Be sure to throw in some physical activities outside the gym, such as tennis, volleyball, golf or any other sport or activity that will keep the blood flowing.

21

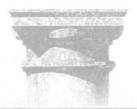

THE ROLE OF DIETARY
SUPPLEMENTATION

I have always been a firm believer that if one continues to treat the symptoms and ignore the root problem, there can only be one result: a greater root problem. Addressing only the symptoms (whether health-related, emotional or spiritual) will cause a person to die prematurely.

If your house were on fire, you would call the fire department. When they arrived, would you prefer that the firefighters hose down the gushing smoke or the fire itself? I hope your answer is the fire!

Regular exercise, eating foods compatible to your blood type and dietary supplementation are the keys for healthy longevity.

Medicating or fighting symptoms after they appear is not the answer. Regular exercise, eating foods compatible to your blood type and dietary supplementation are the keys for healthy longevity. Hormonal control and balance are also necessary for both men and women for a good quality of life.

The Role of Dietary Supplementation

Hormones and Aging

Hormones regulate and influence the functions of the body. As we grow older, our hormone production diminishes, thus causing the appearance of aging. Our bodies lose some of the ability to function as they did when we were young. But we do have the resources that help to prevent this. Aging boomers in search of a more youthful and vibrant entrance into their later years can take supplemental hormones in addition to exercising regularly, eating instinctively and taking general dietary supplements.

The key to slowing down and possibly turning around the symptoms that identify the over-the-hill gang is to bring the body's hormone production back to its normal levels. Age-related diseases, such as heart disease, arthritis, high blood pressure, elevated cholesterol and loss of skin elasticity can be prevented or slowed down by natural hormonal therapy.

The hormones we tend to need as we age are dehydroepiandro-sterone (DHEA), estrogen, testosterone, progesterone, thyroid, insulin, pregnenolone and human growth hormone (HGH).[1] These hormones are all interrelated and must work in harmony to create the synergistic effect required to prevent aging. With a simple saliva test ordered by a physician and some periodical monitoring, you can establish and maintain a hormonal balance in your body.

Aging boomers are able to improve their health and decrease the potential illnesses associated with the aging process by taking supplements to boost their anabolic hormone levels. The question is, When does a person start?

That question reminds me of people trying to decide when to get a face lift. Do they wait until their skin is hanging down to their knees, or do they catch it in the earlier stages? Do you start using HGH or DHEA when you're eighty years old, or do you start when you're fifty? With a visit to see your physician, maybe your best shot at a fountain of youth is right around the corner.

DHEA

Several years ago I made an appointment with a doctor friend of mine to have some blood work done. I wanted to know my blood lipids and my DHEA sulfate levels. I felt good, but work was starting to cause me to drag. I assumed my counts would be normal, but I wanted to check just in case.

When I got my tests back, my level of DHEA sulfate was actually below the low-normal range. That puzzled the doctor and me because typically, when a person takes care of his health as I do, most readings show up in the normal ranges. After discussing my business schedule and the demands on my time, the doctor and I agreed that the low reading was most likely associated with the stress in my life.

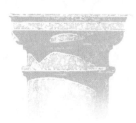

By keeping your DHEA levels up to their maximum, you will help your body be better fit to fight against heart disease, cancers, cardiovascular diseases and obesity.

So he wrote a prescription for DHEA, and I started taking DHEA orally. As I took the supplement, I experienced an improved state of general well-being. I felt somewhat stronger and showed better responses to my training. After one month I went back for another DHEA sulfate test, and this time my level was in the normal range.

It is important to have your DHEA sulfate levels checked through blood testing. DHEA plays a tremendous role in balancing your hormones. This precursor hormone, normally produced in the adrenal glands, is like a conductor of a symphony. It directs the secretions of certain glands to meet the hormonal demands of your body.

When you were in your early twenties, your body had higher levels of DHEA. But as the aging process continued, those levels started to plummet. Though your body was manufacturing 30 milligrams of DHEA at age twenty, unfortunately by age sixty, it only drums up about five milligrams.[2] With the reduction in your body's DHEA levels come the diseases that are associated with getting old.

"When blood levels of DHEA are increased to the level one had at a younger age, many diseases just melt away. The body seems to be fully capable of using supplemental DHEA as if it were processed in the body," says Dr. Julian Whitaker.[3]

By keeping your DHEA levels up to their maximum, you will help your body be better fit to fight against heart disease, cancers, cardiovascular diseases and obesity. Plus, normal levels will assist in creating a hormonal balance among all the hormones listed earlier.

Human growth hormone (HGH)

The increased levels of these major hormones (promoted by normal levels of DHEA) promote the human growth hormone (HGH) production. Human growth hormone is a protein produced in the pituitary gland that stimulates the liver to produce somatomedins, which stimulate growth of bone and muscle. The production of this hormone peaks during adolescence, then steadily declines with age.[4]

HGH levels are at about 400 as a teenager. But, when you arrive at the ripe age of seventy, they are way down to 100.[5] Ask your physician for an IGF-1 (insulin-like growth factor) test. Determining your IGF-1 levels is a way to monitor your HGH levels.

An HGH dietary supplement in pill form is available. But it is ideal to work with your physician to see if you should get on a program of daily injectable HGH.

OTHER LEVELS TO MONITOR

BECAUSE THE LOWERED production of hormones that comes with age has a link to improper fat metabolization, having blood lipids tests

HEALTH **FACT** BOX

POTENTIAL BENEFITS OF HGH THERAPY

- Improved memory
- Improvement of Alzheimer's disease
- Regeneration of the brain, liver and other organs
- Improved sexual function
- Enhanced immunity with increased resistance to infection
- Improved healing of wounds and fractures
- Hair regrowth and color restored
- Improved vision
- Improved exercise tolerance
- Increased muscle mass
- Reduction of fat and cellulite
- Increased energy and stamina
- Increase in HDL (good cholesterol), and decrease in LDL (bad cholesterol)
- Reverse of osteoporosis and strengthening of bones
- Elevation of moods
- Improved sleep patterns
- Improved elasticity and thickness of skin[6]

taken every eighteen months or so is a good idea. This is to monitor your cholesterol levels, the HDL (good cholesterol) and LDL (bad cholesterol) in your blood.

It is also important to monitor levels of homocysteine, an important amino acid used for building particular body proteins.

The Role of Dietary Supplementation

Too high of a level of homocysteine can have a damaging effect on arteries, causing arteriosclerosis and possibly leading to heart attacks and strokes. Some people, regardless of diet, are prone to high levels of homocysteine, which must be controlled.

Your level should not exceed ten, and ideally it should be around seven to eight. Certain B vitamins control homocysteine levels, particularly B_6. This is a water-soluble supplement, so I suggest taking the Recommended Daily Allowance.[7]

ANTIOXIDANTS

MANY INDIVIDUALS SUFFER from pain and illnesses caused by impaired and unbalanced molecules called free radicals. Superoxides, hydroxyl radicals, peroxides and hydroperoxides are examples of free radicals. These impaired molecules attach themselves to healthy cells in the body of the host.

They are not proud invaders; they will settle anywhere. Wherever they attach themselves, they cause a rapid oxidation process, which results in cell damage. If there is free-radical damage to the cells in the walls of the arteries, then plaque buildup is eminent. If cellular damage occurs in the joints due to these culprits, then arthritic pain and discomfort can follow.

Thousands upon thousands of free radicals enter your body every time you inhale the fumes from automobiles, buses and planes. They also affect us when we exercise because we oxidize our cells then.

If you think you can escape them by not going outside or exercising, guess again. Free-radical damage occurs from breathing itself. (Do I have to mention what you would have to do to avoid these guys completely?)

By now almost everyone has heard of antioxidants. These nutrient substances function as scavengers, neutralizing the free-radical molecules. They oppose oxidation and inhibit reactions promoted by oxidation.

211

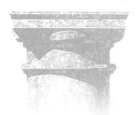

In order for our bodies to continue to function healthfully and energetically, they require a certain amount of attention. The sooner you decide to start giving your body that attention, the sooner you will reap the benefits—more energy, less sickness, more mental alertness, more disease-free living, better mobility, fewer doctor bills, more fun and a greater quality of life.

For example, if there is damage to the lining of the cells in the arterial wall, the antioxidant neutralizes the oxidation action that is destroying the cells and stops the damage. The cells that have not been destroyed can be strengthened by the antioxidant.

Since it is impossible to avoid the attacks of these free radicals, the best thing to do is to defend against them. If you can neutralize their destructive forces and strengthen some of your cells that have been weakened, then you are doing about all you can.

Some antioxidants that can be taken as dietary supplements are vitamin A, vitamin E, selenium, beta carotene, coenzyme Q_{10}, zinc and green tea. Super antioxidants that range from twenty to fifty times the potency of vitamins C and E are called proanthocyanidins. They are generally extracted from the grape seed and are very potent, yet nontoxic.

All antioxidants contribute to strengthening the heart muscles, cleaning the arteries, fighting against cholesterol and cancer and reducing swelling from arthritic pain.

Do your best to avoid the activities that contribute to free radical damage.

START FIGHTING THE AGING PROCESS TODAY

ALL THIS INFORMATION on beating aging might sound too good to be

HEALTH **FACT** BOX

Here are a few other measures you can take to avoid some of the problems associated with free radicals:[8]

- Quit smoking.
- Avoid unsaturated oils, especially the rancid oils often used to deep-fry foods at fast-food restaurants.
- Avoid toxic chemicals as well as toxic fumes from cars and trucks.
- Avoid food additives such as nitrites and nitrates.
- Avoid exposure to x-rays and radiation.

true, but the reality is that many health-conscious people today are already enjoying the benefits of making healthier lifestyle changes as they enter the later years of their lives. In order for our bodies to continue to function healthfully and energetically, they require a certain amount of attention. The sooner you decide to start giving your body that attention, the sooner you will reap the benefits—more energy, less sickness, more mental alertness, more disease-free living, better mobility, fewer doctor bills, more fun and a greater quality of life. It is difficult to break old habits and make new adjustments, but focusing on the end results will keep you on track.

Chronological age does not have to interfere so greatly with the quality of life. Aging adults are becoming more and more aware of the health benefits that come from living an active lifestyle. Subsequently, their chronological age is no longer a factor, limiting them to the premature use of walkers and wheelchairs. Instead, they find themselves experiencing the youthful and energetic lifestyle they did in years prior.

Learning a little more about how your body functions and what it requires to function as it did when you were younger will help you make these lifestyle changes easier. As you begin experiencing the benefits and as your entire life takes on a whole new level of wellness, then you will appreciate how wonderfully your body has been fashioned. Then you can begin to have hope for a healthier and more youthful life as you get older.

God didn't forget a thing when He designed these bodies of ours. The life we live is an extension of our relationship to its Creator. He is the Giver of eternal and physical life. But the responsibility is ours to take control of our lives and do the things that will build up and strengthen our bodies. No one else can do it for us.

As you discover for yourself that the aging process is inevitable, you will realize that the life you are possibly neglecting is the only life you have. Then the issue at hand becomes whether to put forth just a minimum effort or to give it all you have.

Let's not neglect this Pillar. It's not too late to start—but you have to start!

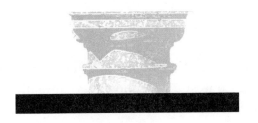

A Word About the One
Who Lives in the Temple

There was a time when everything in my personal and professional life revolved around training, dieting and getting into the best shape I could. Anything else had to fit into my training schedule—vacations, dinners, meetings, even family time. My bodybuilding actually became my god.

That's because I had found a confidence and self-assurance—even my identity—in having larger muscles and hoisting heavier weights. My weight training never failed me the way people did. I always received positive feelings from training. Over the years, the gym had become a place of solitude and safety for me. A driving force within me caused me to train at any hour of the day or night, week in and week out, never missing a workout. For years I put forth tremendous physical effort and dedicated countless hours to building my physical stature. I was a faithful servant to my god.

I pursued wholeness in body, soul and spirit—or so I thought. But the irony of it was that even though I was physically so strong and fit, I still had an area of great weakness in my life. I thought I could recklessly abandon one area of my makeup, expecting somehow to obtain a balance by overdoing another.

At first I didn't realize a weakness existed. But as it grew, the recognition of it floated from my subconscious up to my conscious mind. It was like an emptiness, a deep loneliness, a longing too strong for words.

215

Seven Pillars of Health

All the while I was increasing in strength physically. I won bodybuilding contests. My body was certainly showing the benefits of exercise and diet, and my mind was strong and confident. But the awareness of that void grew, and nothing I tried filled it.

I know now why I couldn't fill that emptiness. It is impossible for human beings to mend the spiritual part of themselves that is lacking in true life. Man can't reach up and touch God. But God can reach down and touch man. And He reached down and touched me.

In 1984 I felt that touch for the first time. I knelt beside my bed in my little apartment and talked to the God I had heard about in Sunday school decades before. I told Him that I was tired of my life, tired of my emptiness and my feeble and destructive attempts to fill it. And He took me just as I was.

This new spirituality was not at all like the wholeness I thought I had attained by "balancing" my body, soul and spirit. This was much deeper than simple acts of kindness, thoughtfulness and respect shown toward others. It was much more than that feeling of well-being and satisfaction in being fit. I could finally see that all those things were of human origin and filled with human limitations.

But what I experienced was not of human origin. This man of iron had to humble himself and admit his need in order to have the Giver of life touch and heal him. Then I was brought to a true wholeness of body, soul and spirit. Admitting my limitations brought His limitlessness into my life.

This true wholeness in body, soul and spirit would have been impossible without supernatural regeneration through His Spirit.

After I experienced this new spiritual birth, my perspective toward physical fitness changed radically. My former god was replaced by God in heaven. Jesus became the center of my life.

A Word About the One Who Lives in the Temple

Since then, I have come to the understanding that I have a higher calling. God has allowed me to keep the fitness orientation that was once my god, but now I use it as a platform to serve Him.

God has taught me that He is the Giver of both physical and spiritual life, which has given me a greater appreciation of how much He cares. I have eternal life to experience with Him when this life on earth passes. I have absolutely nothing to lose, but everything to gain.

The Bible teaches that my body is the temple of the Spirit of God. That means His Spirit lives within me. So now, my attitude about training, dieting, taking supplements and using preventative measures to live a healthier life has become a *spiritual issue.* By doing the things that will promote a better quality of physical life (and avoiding those things that hinder it), I'm being a faithful caretaker of this temple. And I do that so I will have the strength and stamina to accomplish what He desires while I'm on this earth.

I have found a deeper reason for keeping my body in shape, and this higher calling requires commitment and constancy—not for my own benefit alone, but so I am able to function physically and mentally at my best for His glory. Psychologically and emotionally, I have renewed strength because I have discovered I can turn all my problems and concerns to Him, and He always gives me peace.

If you want true balance in your body, soul and spirit, then trust Jesus as your Savior. You need Him! Don't miss out. He will fill the void in your life—the one you may not even know is there until He fills it.

God shows His love toward all humans through His Son, Jesus. His love was demonstrated by laying His life down as our substitute, thereby removing the consequences and punishment for our wrongdoings. Through being sorry for what we have done and turning from it, then believing that He and He alone provides an eternal home in His family for us, we can become truly alive spiritually.

Let Him take charge of you—body, soul and spirit. Ask Him now to take you as His own and give you eternal life. He promised that to anyone who would ask Him.

As you strengthen your Pillars of Health, let your primary focus be the One living in your temple with you. Get to know your loving heavenly Father through His Son, Jesus.

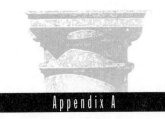

Eating For
Your Blood Type

I f you desire more detailed information on eating for your blood type, I recommend the book I have co-authored with Dr. Steven M. Weissberg, M.D., *The Answer Is in Your Blood-type*. It is reader friendly and full of information, including pages of foods, from meats to condiments and spices, for each blood type. Beneficial foods, neutral foods and foods to avoid are each listed separately for each blood type. Included also are sample 7-day menu plans for each blood type.

For further information on how to order *The Answer Is in Your Bloodtype* or specific dietary supplements for your blood type, contact us:

PERSONAL NUTRITION USA
P. O. Box 951479 • Lake Mary, Florida 32795
Phone: 1-888-41Blood
E-mail to: Bloodtype2@aol.com
Web site: www.4blood.com

For information on the colon cleanse, dietary supplements for fibromyalgia, chronic fatigue syndrome, energy boosters, exercise equipment and exercise videos, contact us:

BODY REDESIGNING
P. O. Box 951479 • Lake Mary, Florida 32795
Phone: 1-800-259-BODY
Email: jac10@aol.com
Web site: www.bodyredesigning.com

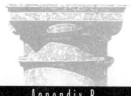

CALCULATING YOUR EXERCISE
TARGET HEART RATE

The example given below is for a forty-year-old person.

1. Determine your true resting heart rate by taking your pulse when you wake up in the morning while you are still in bed. (As your cardiovascular condition improves, you will notice a lower resting heart rate.) Take your pulse at the carotid artery on the neck, immediately to the right or left of the Adam's apple. Touch it with the index and middle finger to feel the pulse. Count the heart beats for 30 seconds and multiply by 2 to get beats per minute.

   Example: Resting heart rate = 64 beats per minute.

2. Calculate your maximal heart rate.
   Maximal heart rate = 220 − age.
   Example: 220 − 40 = 180 beats per minute

3. Calculate heart rate reserve.
   Heart rate reserve = Maximal heart rate − resting heart rate
   Example: 180 − 64 = 116 beats per minute

   4. Determine the work intensity range.
   Work intensity range = heart rate reserve x percent intensity
   Example: For 70 percent intensity range (aerobic training level), 116 x 70% (.70) = 81

5. Add back in resting heart rate.
   Example: 70 + 64 = 135 beats per minute
   81 + 64 = 145 beats per minute

Calculating Your Exercise Target Heart Rate

Here is a condensed version of the above example:

220 − 40 = 180
180 − 64 = 116
116 x .70 = 81
81 + 64 = 145 beats per minute

When you are checking your heart rate during exercise, take your pulse for 10 seconds and multiply it by 6. Example: 23 beats x 10 seconds = 138 beats per minute.

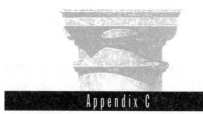

WALKING PROGRAM CHART

1. Begin slowly.

2. Wear proper shoes (i.e., Rockport or Reebok Walkers).

3. Do not progress to the next level until you are comfortable.

4. Monitor your heart rate, and stay within your target range.

5. Listen to your body. Be aware of new aches or pains.

6. Drink plenty of water when exercising in the heat.

7. Don't walk in heat of 90 degrees or in humidity of 80 percent. Be careful.

8. Take a pulse check at the half-way point and end of each walk.

Walking Program Chart

DAY	DURATION	DISTANCE	HEART RATE	HOW DO YOU FEEL?
1	20 minutes	_____	1___ 2___	_____
2	20 minutes	_____	1___ 2___	_____
3	20 minutes	_____	1___ 2___	_____
4	20 minutes	_____	1___ 2___	_____
5	25 minutes	_____	1___ 2___	_____
6	25 minutes	_____	1___ 2___	_____
7	25 minutes	_____	1___ 2___	_____
8	25 minutes	_____	1___ 2___	_____
9	30 minutes	_____	1___ 2___	_____
10	35 minutes	_____	1___ 2___	_____
11	35 minutes	_____	1___ 2___	_____
12	35 minutes	_____	1___ 2___	_____
13	35 minutes	_____	1___ 2___	_____
14	45 minutes	_____	1___ 2___	_____
15	45 minutes	_____	1___ 2___	_____
16	45 minutes	_____	1___ 2___	_____
17	45 minutes	_____	1___ 2___	_____
18	45 minutes	_____	1___ 2___	_____
19	50 minutes	_____	1___ 2___	_____
20	50 minutes	_____	1___ 2___	_____
21	50 minutes	_____	1___ 2___	_____
22	50 minutes	_____	1___ 2___	_____
23	50 minutes	_____	1___ 2___	_____
24	55 minutes	_____	1___ 2___	_____
25	55 minutes	_____	1___ 2___	_____
26	55 minutes	_____	1___ 2___	_____
27	55 minutes	_____	1___ 2___	_____
28	55 minutes	_____	1___ 2___	_____
29	60 minutes	_____	1___ 2___	_____
30	60 minutes	_____	1___ 2___	_____

**When you get to 60 minutes, or before if you like, try to walk the same distance, decreasing your time. Remember to stay within your target heart rate.

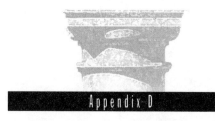

GLYCEMIC INDEX

Some carbs enter the bloodstream more rapidly than others and can quickly be utilized for energy. The chart beow compares foods containing carbs in terms of their effect on blood sugar, using a scale on which glucose rates 100.

The best foods to eat before high-endurance exercise, such as a marathon, long-distance running or exercising one hour or more in duration, are found in the low glycemic index (less than 40). The best foods to eat after a shorter, more intense exercise, like sprinting or weight-training, should come from the high glycemic index (above 60).

Be sure to choose carefully and aim for variety in these foods.

HIGH (PROVIDES FAST ENERGY)		MODERATE		LOW (SUSTAINED ENERGY)	
Potato, baked	.85	Bran Chex	.58	Apple	.36
Corn flakes	.84	Orange juice	.57	Pear	.36
Rice cakes	.82	Rice, white long-grain	.56	Chocolate milk	.34
Cheerios	.74	Rice, brown	.55	Fruit yogurt, low-fat	.33
Crem of Wheat, instant	.74	Corn	.55	Chickpeas	.33
Graham crackers	.74	Sweet potato	.54	Lima beans, frozen	.32
Watermelon	.72	Banana, overripe	.52	Milk, skim	.32
Bagel, white	.72	Peas, green	.48	Apricots, dry	.31
Bread, whole wheat	.69	Baked beans	.48	Green beans	.30
Shredded wheat	.69	Lentil soup	.44	Banana, under ripe	.30
Grape-nuts	.67	Orange	.43	Lentils	.29
Stoned wheat thins	.67	All-Bran cereal	.42	Kidney beans	.27
Cream of Wheat, regular	.66	Spaghetti (no sauce)	.41	Milk, whole	.27
Couscous	.65	Pumpernickel bread	.41	Barley	.25
Raisins	.64	Apple juice, unsweetened	.41	Grapefruit	.25
Oatmeal	.61				
Bran muffin	.60				

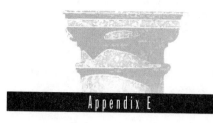

YOUR
EXERCISE JOURNAL

	A.M.	P.M.
Time of Workout	____	____

Workout	Yes	No
Strength Training	____	____
Aerobic Exercise	____	____

Length of Workout	Hrs.	Min.
Strength Training	____	____
Aerobic Exercise	____	____

Monitor Heart Rate

Aerobic _____ bpm (beats per minute)

Comments (how you felt before and after workout, improvements in energy, strength, etc.):

_____

_____

_____

Feedback received:

_____

_____

_____

Rewards:

_____

_____

_____

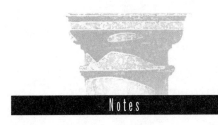

Notes

INTRODUCTION

1. Albert Zehr, Ph.D., *Healthy Steps to Maintain or Regain Natural Good Health* (Burnaby, Canada: Abundant Health Publishers, 1990), 34.

CHAPTER 2
WEIGHT AND THE PERFECT BODY

1. Karen M. Carrier, "Breaking Out of the Dieting Prison," *Health and Fitness Idea Source,* February 1998, 5.

CHAPTER 3
WEIGHT AND YOUR HEALTH

1. Source obtained from the Internet: "Statistics Related to Overweight and Obesity," National Institute of Diabetes and Digestive and Kidney Diseases (NIDDK), www.niddk.nih.gov/health/nutrit/pubs/statobes.htm.
2. Rob Wilkins and Mike O'Hearn, "Obesity! Public Enemy Number One," *Natural Muscle Magazine,* January 2000, 28.
3. Ibid.
4. Ibid.
5. Ibid.
6. Associated Press, "Government order—exercise," *The Orlando Sentinel,* January 26, 2000, A-3.
7. Wilkins and O'Hearn, "Obesity! Public Enemy Number One," 28.
8. Ibid.
9. Ibid.

10. Ibid.
11. Source obtained from the Internet: www.weight.com/definition.html.
12. Source obtained from the Internet: Michael Blumenkrantz, "Obesity: The World's Oldest Metabolic Disorder," www.quantumhcp.com/ obesity.htm.
13. Wilkins and O'Hearn, "Obesity! Public Enemy Number One," 29.
14. Blumenkrantz, "Obesity: The World's Oldest Metabolic Disorder."
15. Wilkins and O'Hearn, "Obesity! Public Enemy Number One," 29–30.
16. "Statistics Related to Overweight and Obesity," National Institute of Diabetes and Digestive and Kidney Diseases.
17. Source obtained from the Internet: www.4BetterHealth.com

CHAPTER 4

THE DESPAIR OF DIETING

1. Statistics compiled from the following Internet sources: "Statistics and Research," www.medicalinvestment.com/quotesandstatistics.html; www.caloriecontrol.org/dietfigs.html; and www.aomc.org/HOD2/ general/weight-DIET.html.

CHAPTER 5

THE BLOOD TYPE CONNECTION TO DIET

1. Source obtained from the Internet: "Hypoglycemia," National Diabetes Information Clearing House, www.niddk.nih.gov/health/diabetes/ pubs/hypo/hypo.htm.

CHAPTER 7

ELIMINATION—THE UNMENTIONABLE SUBJECT

1. Zehr, *Healthy Steps to Maintain or Regain Natural Good Health*, 34.
2. Source obtained from the Internet: The Intestinal System, www.webcom.com/drweed/systems.

Notes

3. Zehr, *Healthy Steps to Maintain or Regain Natural Good Health*, 35.
4. Ibid.
5. Ibid.
6. Ibid., 38.
7. Ibid.
8. Source obtained from Internet: The Intestinal System, ww.webcom.com.
9. Zehr, *Healthy Steps to Maintain or Regain Natural Good Health*, 39.
10. Ibid., 41.
11. Ibid.

CHAPTER 8
INVASION OF THE PARASITES

1. Teresa Schumacher and Toni Schumacher Lund, *Cleansing the Body and the Colon for a Happier and Healthier You* (n.p., 1987), 10.
2. Ibid.
3. Dolly Katz, *Miami Herald,* quoted in Schumacher and Lund, *Cleansing the Body and the Colon for a Happier and Healthier You,* 10.
4. Schumacher and Lund, *Cleansing the Body and the Colon for a Happier and Healthier You,* 10.
5. Ibid., 13.
6. Ibid., 11.
7. Ibid., 26.
8. Ibid., 15.
9. Ibid., 14.

CHAPTER 9
CLEANSING THE COLON

1. Pamela Smith, *Eat Well–Live Well* (Lake Mary, FL: Creation House, 1992), 39.
2. Joseph Christiano, *Back to Basics Nutrition Manual* (Lake Mary, FL: LOJO Productions, Inc., 1993).

3. Source obtained from the Internet: "Just the Fats, Ma'am," www.phys.com/d_magazines/01self/fats/basic4.htm.
4. Schumacher and Lund, *Cleansing the Body and Colon for a Happier and Healthier You,* 28.

CHAPTER 10
THE IMMUNE SYSTEM: ARMED FORCES AGAINST INVADERS

1. Source obtained from the Internet: Normal Lymphocytes, www.mcL.tulane.edu.

CHAPTER 11
ENEMY INFILTRATORS

1. Dr. Peter J. D'Adamo, with Catherine Whitney, *Eat Right for Your Type* (New York: G. P. Putnam's Sons, 1996).
2. Source obtained from the Internet: Stewart B. Levy, "The Challenge of Antibiotic Resistance," www.sciam.com/1998/0398issue/0398Levy.html.
3. Lisa Landymore-Lim, *Poisonous Prescriptions* (Subraco, WA, Australia: PODD, 1994).
4. Zehr, *Healthy Steps to Maintain or Regain Natural Good Health,* 58.
5. Source obtained from the Internet: "Innovations in Cancer Therapy," www.bu.edu.cohis/cancer/about/innoutx.htm.

CHAPTER 12
KEEPING THE IMMUNE ARMY STRONG

1. Zehr, *Healthy Steps to Maintain or Regain Natural Good Health,* 59.
2. Source obtained from the Internet: "Fibromyalgia," www.intelihealth.com.
3. Ibid.

CHAPTER 13
THE BENEFITS OF EXERCISE

1. Source obtained from the Internet: www.state.id.us/dhw/hwgd_www/ health/hp/part_2.pdf.

Notes

2. Associated Press, "Government order—exercise," *The Orlando Sentinel,* January 26, 2000, A–3.

CHAPTER 16
THE IMPORTANCE OF R AND R

1. Source obtained from the Internet: "Managing Stress—Part III: Too Much of Good Thing?", Mental Health resources, http://mentalhealth.miningco.com/health/mentalhealth/libra ry/weekly/aa0082498.htm.

CHAPTER 17
PROGRESSIVE RELAXATION

1. Adapted from the *HFI Workbook,* American College of Sports and Medicine, and *Stress Management Training Program,* Adelphi University.

CHAPTER 18
A GOOD NIGHT'S REST

1. Charles W. Rice, Jr., "Sleep Deprivation…Your Worst Nightmare!", *Natural Muscle Magazine,* November 1999, 67.
2. Ibid.
3. Zehr, *Healthy Steps to Maintain or Regain Natural Good Health,* 109.
4. Ibid., 110.
5. James F. Balch, M.D., and Phyllis A. Balch, C.N.C., *Prescription for Nutritional Healing* (Garden City Park, NY: Avery Publishers Group, 1997), 72.
6. Zehr, *Healthy Steps to Maintain or Regain Natural Good Health,* 112.

CHAPTER 19
AGING AND DETERIORATION

1. Ken Dychtwalk, "Baby Boomers Ready to Get Fit," quoted in Lisa Johnson, "Boomers Bloom," *American Fitness,* November/December 1996, 45.
2. Jeff Ostroff, *Successful Marketing to the 50+ Consumer,*

quoted in Lisa Johnson, "Boomers Bloom," *American Fitness,* November/December 1996, 45.

3. Terrie Heinrich Rizzo, MAS, and Karl Knopf, Ed.D., "Resistance Training for Older Adults," *Health and Fitness Idea Source,* June 1999, 33.
4. Ibid.
5. Source obtained from the Internet: Bill Burkart, "Marketers Must View Boomers Through a New Lens," www.neoa.org/news/archives/marketers_view.html.
6. Ibid.
7. Lisa Johnson, "Boomers Bloom," *American Fitness,* November/ December 1996, 47.
8. Source obtained from the Internet: www.medicine-antiaging.com/ test.htm.
9. Rizzo and Knopf, "Resistance Training for Older Adults."
10. Ibid.
11. Ibid.
12. Ibid.
13. Ibid., 34.

CHAPTER 20
BEATING THE AGING PROCESS WITH EXERCISE

1. Source obtained from the Internet: Mark S. Lander, "Turning Back Time With Exercise," America Online: Bloodtype 2, copyright © 2000 by iVillage, Inc.
2. Johnson, "Boomers Bloom," 47.
3. Ibid., 45.
4. Source obtained from the Internet: "Living to the Max," *Modern Maturity,* July/August 1999, www.aarp.org.
5. Ibid.

CHAPTER 21
THE ROLE OF DIETARY SUPPLEMENTATION

1. Source obtained from the Internet: R. W. Noble, M.D., diplomat of the American Board of Anti-Aging Medicine, "What is Anti-Aging Medicine?", www.medicine-antiaging.com.

Notes

2. "Nutrition's Newest Discovery: DHEA," *Amazing Discovery* pamphlet, January 1995.
3. Julian Whitaker, *Health and Healing* (n.p., n.d.), quoted in *Amazing Discovery* pamphlet, January 1995.
4. Source obtained from the Internet: Glossary of Terms Related to HGH (Human Growth Hormone), www.vibrantforlife.com.
5. Source obtained from the Internet: www.medicine-antiaging.com/ test.htm.
6. Source obtained from the Internet: R. W. Noble, M.D., diplomat of the American Board of Anti-Aging Medicine, "What Is Anti-Aging Medicine?", www.medicine-antiaging.com/test.htm.
7. Ibid.
8. Zehr, *Healthy Steps to Maintain or Regain Natural Good Health*, 103.

You can feel better,
BE BETTER!
You're finding new
health, vitality and
strength in your body.
How about your spirit?

If you'd like more information on how you can live "healthy"—body, soul *and* spirit—call, e-mail or write us. SILOAM PRESS offers a wealth of resources on how to eat better, exercise better, feel better, LIVE BETTER.

www.creationhouse.com
fax: 407-333-7100
Toll-free information line—
1-800-599-5750

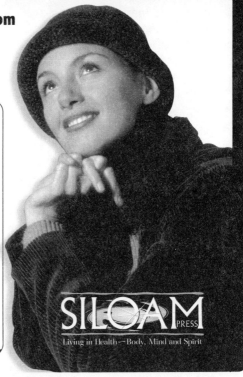

We've got a wealth of trustworthy resources. Call us for a **free catalog** or more information on—

○ Nutrition
○ Alternative medicine
○ Diet
○ Spiritual growth
○ Healthy recipes
○ Mental & emotional growth
○ Fighting cancer & other diseases
○ Healthy relationships

SILOAM PRESS
Living in Health—Body, Mind and Spirit

Your Walk With God Can Be Even Deeper...

With *Charisma* magazine, you'll be informed and inspired by the features and stories about what the Holy Spirit is doing in the lives of believers today.

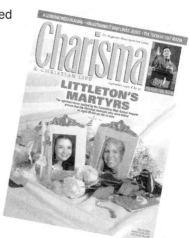

Each issue:

- Brings you exclusive world-wide reports to rejoice over.
- Keeps you informed on the latest news from a Christian perspective.
- Includes miracle-filled testimonies to build your faith.
- Gives you access to relevant teaching and exhortation from the most respected Christian leaders of our day.

Call 1-800-829-3346 for 3 FREE trial issues
Offer #AOACHB

If you like what you see, then pay the invoice of $22.97 (**saving over 51% off the cover price**) and receive 9 more issues (12 in all). Otherwise, write "cancel" on the invoice, return it, and owe nothing.

Experience the Power of Spirit-Led Living

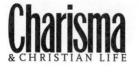

Charisma Offer #AOACHB
P.O. Box 420234
Palm Coast, Florida 32142-0234
www.charismamag.com